PENGUIN BOOKS

# HEADACHES AND MIGRAINE

Shirley Trickett is a former nurse who has worked in the community for fourteen years, encouraging people to take responsibility for their own physical, emotional and spiritual health. Her methods are simple and can be used with the conventional medical help the person is already receiving.

She is the author of *Coming Off Tranquillizers and Sleeping Pills* (Thorsons, 1986), *Coping with Anxiety and Depression* (Sheldon, 1989), *The Irritable Bowel Syndrome and Diverticulosis* (Thorsons, 1990), *Coping Successfully with Panic Attacks* (Sheldon, 1992), *Coping with Candida: Are Yeast Infections Draining Your Energy?* (Sheldon, 1994) and *The Candida Cookbook* (Thorsons, 1995). Her books are simple and practical, and are used by the public, by GPs and in hospitals. In 1987 she won a Whitbread Community Care Award.

Shirley Trickett is a widow with two daughters, a son and three grandchildren. She lives in north-east England.

'Once again Shirley has written a gem of a book, full of easy to understand facts and practical tips on the management of this very common but often difficult to treat problem. Like her previous titles, I will have no hesitation in recommending this book to both my patients and colleagues. I cannot wait for the next one' – Dr A. J. Wright, MBChB, DRCOG, MRCGP

**SHIRLEY TRICKETT**

*Headaches and Migraine*

*Understand the Causes and Take Control with This
Complete Guide to Pain Prevention and Relief*

PENGUIN BOOKS

PENGUIN BOOKS

Published by the Penguin Group
Penguin Books Ltd, 27 Wrights Lane, London w8 5tz, England
Penguin Books USA Inc., 375 Hudson Street, New York, New York 10014, USA
Penguin Books Australia Ltd, Ringwood, Victoria, Australia
Penguin Books Canada Ltd, 10 Alcorn Avenue, Toronto, Ontario, Canada m4v 3b2
Penguin Books (NZ) Ltd, 182–190 Wairau Road, Auckland 10, New Zealand

Penguin Books Ltd, Registered Offices: Harmondsworth, Middlesex, England

First published 1996
10 9 8 7 6 5 4 3 2 1

Set in 11/13.75 pt Monotype Bembo
Typeset by RefineCatch Limited, Bungay, Suffolk
Printed in England by Clays Ltd, St Ives plc

For my twin sister Sheila and her
husband Henricus, the love and support of whom
has saved me many a 'headache'

# CONTENTS

# LIST OF FIGURES

# INTRODUCTION

---

In headaches and worry life leaks away
W. H. AUDEN

For the past twelve years I have worked with the public teaching self-help methods for relief of all types of pain, sore heads, aching shoulders, backs tight with muscle spasm, the pain of drug addiction, the pain of loss and, perhaps hardest of all to witness, depression, the pain of loss of self. Pain hurts – it's meant to – it alerts us to the fact that something is wrong, that we must act.

Common headaches respond well to self-help methods and there are several avenues suggested in this book for you to explore to discover why you are having headaches. There are also many practical measures given for relieving your symptoms.

## Working towards Wholeness

Release from pain often brings the energy necessary for change. Is it time for you to stop 'beating yourself with sticks': I should do this, I should do that? Is it time for you to discover who you really are, to find your own truth and not be contented with the fake picture of self you have come to accept – a collage of impressions built up initially from feedback from parents/siblings/teachers and, in your adult life, from what your partner/boss/friends and others say you are?

## *Allowing Yourself as Long as It Takes*

Taking the time to discover what is causing your headaches could also be the time for taking a compassionate look at yourself and perhaps looking at 'the pain beyond the pain' – the suppressed aspects of self, your deep needs and desires – a time for retaining only the learning from past emotional pain and letting go of the rest.

## *Acceptance of Who You Are*

Until you accept that you are a special being worthy of self-respect and love it is unlikely that you will find the inner peace necessary to work towards true health – the harmonious interaction of body, mind, emotions and spirit. As feelings of self-worth grow so will your confidence, and as old fears recede the crutches of addictions, obsessions, overdependence on relationships and work can be discarded, and as you love yourself and become centred in your being you can continue on your chosen path with a much lighter step.

'Love is the highest degree of medicine' – PARACELSUS

SHIRLEY TRICKETT

PART ONE

# Headaches and Migraines

# I

# *The Volcano Effect*

It is unlikely that your headache will have a single precipitating factor. Chronic headaches can be the end result of a long chain of events. You might have been laying the foundation stones for your headaches for many years, possibly since childhood, even since birth, with that first monumental headache that was necessary for your entry into the world.

## The Smouldering Volcano

Think of your body as a volcano, a baseline of seismic activity. The smouldering comes from your physical, emotional and spiritual reactions to your life circumstances, which provide a continual background of strain. It then only needs a trigger for it to explode into a full-blown eruption – your headache.

## What is the Function of a Headache?

Your body, far from letting you down when it produces a headache, is trying to make you aware of how harshly you are treating it, and it will continue to plague you with pain until you listen. It is trying to make you change some aspect, or possibly more than one destructive pattern of behaviour – trying to get you to stop and *think*.

## A Headache Enforces Rest

It might be saying to you: why do you continually overwork/
when are you going to look to your emotional needs/when are
you going to eat sensibly/when are you going to cut down on
alcohol/when are you going to get out of that relationship/
when are you going to realize your immune system is very
low/when are you going to follow your life purpose? The list is
endless.

## Beginning at the Beginning

Many people understandably become obsessed by the headache
but fail to see it as an end result, not the start of their problems or
how they are treating their body. 'If only I did not get these
headaches life would be wonderful.' This is unlikely; headaches
don't evolve without favourable conditions and, in any case, if
you did not get headaches nature might prod you in some other
way to force you to take stock. It could be by giving you digestive problems, panic attacks, asthma, depression or any chronic
condition which forces you temporarily to slow down. Which
condition manifests in you will depend on where your weak
spot is. Have you noticed that when a long-term stress-induced
malady for some reason disappears *there is always another one standing in the queue ready to take its place*? Perhaps this is the body
saying, 'Well if you won't listen to what a gastric ulcer is telling
you let's try panic attacks – they can lead to agoraphobia and
then see if you can carry on working at this pace!'

All recurrent conditions highlight the fact that your being is
not balanced, is not in harmony. This is the baseline. This is
where your detective work begins, taking an honest look at what
is smouldering at the bottom of your volcano and being open
enough to admit that whatever is lurking there is your responsibility, not your doctor's (providing, of course, that he has fully

investigated your symptoms). Nor are they the fault of your boss/partner/mother-in-law. You cannot change their behaviour no matter how unreasonable it is. All you have control over is your reaction to your position – how much you are going to allow yourself to be affected and, in short, how much you are going to stoke the fires of your volcano.

## But My Headaches are Purely Physical

You might want to protest, 'But it is only stuffy rooms/sinus problems/sunlight/loud noise and so on that affect me. It is physical.' If you read section . . . you will see that nothing can be 'just physical' – the autonomic nervous system is governed by the emotions, which in turn affect the circulation, the muscles, the immune system and so on, and although this may be a bit esoteric for some, I believe that the emotions depend on the spirit. So everything affects everything else. If you find all this discouraging and wonder where to start, remember that the good news is, because of this interdependency, any positive actions towards balance in one area will affect the whole being.

# 2

# List of Suspects

This book aims to encourage headache sufferers to turn detective and discover what is causing their headaches. The holistic, active role is stressed and it is hoped that sufferers will be excited by the opportunity to participate in their own improved health or cure. Headaches are rarely fatal, but they can cause great distress, not only because they can be such agony but also because they can destroy self-esteem and the ability to cope. They can also be responsible for loss of employment and loss of relationships, and lead to suicidal depression.

The book describes different types of headaches, lists common causes and discusses a variety of simple self-help treatments. It presupposes that the reader's symptoms have been investigated by his/her doctor, that a firm diagnosis has been made and that the type of headache diagnosed falls into the group which responds well to self-help methods. This group includes tension headaches, migraine, allergic headaches and many more, as you will see when you read on.

## What is a Headache?

A headache is a pain in the head which can range from a slight ache that makes life a bit dreary, but does not seriously affect concentration, to a pain so disabling that the thought process is severely disturbed and the sufferer is completely prostrate. The degree of pain is usually determined by the amount of swelling in the soft tissue of the head. It is easy to see why this can be so agonizing: if your arm needed to swell it is free to do so, but since the brain is confined by the bony case of the skull there is no relief until the swelling subsides. Common descriptions of headaches suggest this pressure: 'I thought my head would split', 'I felt as though my head was in a vice.'

## What is a Headache Saying?

A headache is the head saying that you are subjecting it to conditions it cannot tolerate. A mild headache may be saying, 'Can't you do something about this?'; a severe headache caused by poisonous fumes may be saying 'Get out of here, your life is in danger.'

Headaches don't descend on us without reason and you may have to accept that, however unwittingly, you are actually causing yours. This will become clearer as you understand the needs of the head:

normal circulation
nourishment
the correct balance of oxygen and carbon dioxide
absence of toxic substances.

In a healthy person it is unlikely that a headache would develop if these needs are met.

# COMMON HEADACHES

| | |
|---|---|
| *Tension* | Caused by contraction of the muscles |
| *Migraine* | Caused by altered circulation to the head |
| *Hormonal* | Caused by changing hormone levels, for |

|  | example, premenstrual tension, the menopause, taking the pill |
|---|---|
| *Post-stress* | Caused by dilation of blood vessels after period of constriction |
| *Allergic* | Caused by exposure to pollens, moulds, chemicals, foods |
| *Infective* | Caused by bacteria or viruses |
| *Structural* | Caused by bones being out of alignment, for example the jaw bone |
| *Postural* | Caused by putting a strain on the muscles of the head, neck and shoulders |
| *Eye strain* | Caused by overuse of the muscles around the eyes |
| *Hypoglycaemic* | Caused by rapid changes in the blood sugar levels; dieting, poor nutrition, irregular meals |
| *Toxic* | Caused by overindulgence in food and drink, constipation, absorption of toxins from the colon |
| *Drug-induced* | Caused either by ingestion of drugs or as part of the withdrawal reaction |
| *Hyperventilation* | Caused by an unbalanced mixture of oxygen and carbon dioxide in the brain |
| *Atmospheric* | Caused by geopathic stress—gases, radiation, positive ions, stuffy rooms |
| *Electrical pollution* | Caused by power cables, VDUs, etc. |

# WHICH TYPE OF HEADACHE?

There are two main types of headache and if you can decide which one plagues you, then the causes will be easier to pinpoint and it will be easier to find effective treatment.

## Tight-muscle (Tension) Headaches

This is the most common type of headache. When muscles in the head, neck or shoulders are shortened (contracted), blood vessels are constricted and the circulation to the brain is affected. The neck is the gateway to the head and if this gate is partially closed the results are dull headaches, woolly thinking, dizziness and irritability. Many sufferers from this type of headache are unaware of the extent of the congestion in their muscles until firm pressure around the base of the skull, the back of the neck or the shoulders causes them to howl in protest. When the blood circulates freely the waste products of metabolism (the burning of the food we eat) are rinsed away and excreted. When the muscles are tight the waste products are trapped and form crystals. It is when these are pressed on to the bones that the pain is felt. If you are tender in these muscles and your headache is relieved by a head and shoulder massage, you can be fairly sure it is a *tight-muscle or tension headache*. Alcohol is a powerful muscle relaxant so if your symptoms are improved by a drink, this could confirm the diagnosis.

### Appearance of Person with Tension Headache

If the blood vessels are dilated the face can be flushed or puffy and the eyes bloodshot. If the blood vessels are contracted the face is usually pale. One or both shoulders can be pulled up towards the ears, the head can be inclined to one side or the chin may be jutting forward in the turtle position. Why this happens will be explained later. Lying flat can increase blood flow to the head and relieve symptoms. Muscular headaches can be caused by stress, trauma, posture, allergies, infections, low body temperature and low blood sugar. Sometimes it is not just one factor but a combination that starts a headache.

## Dilated-blood-vessel (Vascular) Headaches

The pain in this type of headache is usually caused by pressure on the nerves as the blood vessels swell. Migraine and hormonal headaches, such as those experienced premenstrually and during the menopause, could be in this group. Alcohol and lying flat, because they increase blood flow to the head, usually make the symptoms worse.

### Appearance of Person with Vascular Headache

If the blood vessels are dilated the face can be flushed or puffy and the eyes bloodshot. If the blood vessels are contracted the face is usually pale.

## Combination Headaches

You may get different types of headaches at different times or sometimes you may feel you have a mixture of the two types. The pain from a vascular headache can cause you to tighten head and neck muscles and so compound the problem.

# IT'S *YOUR* HEAD

If your doctor has ruled out conditions which would cause headaches such as high blood pressure, and you have recently had your eyes tested, it is really up to you to discover what you are doing in your daily routine to make your head object so strongly. Some people become angry when their doctor cannot reveal the cause of their headaches, and feel discouraged when they leave the surgery with yet another prescription for painkillers. They are often reluctant to take these, either because they don't find them very effective or because they feel they have been on drugs for too long. If you feel angry with your doctor, try to remember that he is probably not disputing that you have headaches, only that he is baffled by the cause. Don't be worried by the diagnosis 'ideopathic headaches'; this only means headaches of unknown origin. After you have read the next chapters (and always assuming that your doctor has ruled out any serious disorder), you will see that it makes more sense for you to be the sleuth because he/she cannot know enough about your life to pinpoint one of the multitude of causes.

Tension and vascular headaches will be looked at in more detail in Chapters 5 and 6. The next chapter alerts you to some medical emergencies.

**3**

# When to Call the Doctor

*Headaches Which Need Urgent or Continued*
*Medical Attention*

**Medical instructions must be followed at all times. Do not cut
down or stop medication or change your treatment in any
way without consulting your doctor.**

Having said that, there are many headaches where self-help
methods enhance the conventional medical treatment. For example, if you have severe sinusitis and need an antibiotic, using
steam inhalations or essential oils as well can reduce swelling and
ease pain, and taking supplements which will stop the antibiotics
upsetting your digestion or giving you thrush can only be of
value. The other great benefit of self-help is learning what to do
to prevent further attacks (prophylactic treatment). For example,
if you understand that depleting your immune system is asking
for repeated infections and you take steps to correct this, it could
turn you from a passive prescription-taker to a person who has
enough knowledge to avoid or limit further attacks.

## WHEN TO SEEK MEDICAL HELP

### After Injury

Headaches after injury should always be investigated even if the
onset is some time after the injury. This does not mean you need

to rush off to the doctor every time your child bumps its head, but if the colour does not return to the face of the child (or adult), and there is vomiting, drowsiness, irritability or loss of consciousness, seek urgent help. It could be that there is increased pressure in the brain (intracranial) due to swelling or bleeding.

## Any Sudden Severe Headache

Unless the person is a known headache sufferer where the cause has been established and the symptoms are the same as in previous attacks, seek help. Known headache sufferers, say a person who has tension headaches or migraine, are not immune from other causes of severe headaches such as strokes.

## Known Headache Sufferers

If the nature of the headache changes in frequency or severity, if the usual treatment affords no relief or if the pain is accompanied by any new symptoms, including:

    blackouts
    dizziness
    visual disturbances
    speech difficulties: either difficulty making the tongue work
        properly or inability to remember words
    clumsiness
    muscle weakness or numbness
    incontinence
    depression

seek help and explain any new symptoms to the doctor. He/she might want to review diagnosis and treatment.

## Don't Panic

If you have developed any symptoms which your doctor does not know about or any of the above symptoms, you should seek medical attention, but there is no need to panic and assume you have some serious illness. The same symptoms can be found in many conditions such as migraine, drug withdrawal and severe anxiety.

## Prescribed Drugs

If you have been given new medication for any condition and you develop headaches, consult your doctor. Headaches are a side-effect of many drugs and you may be told that they are to be expected and will ease off as your body adjusts to the drug. If, however, the headaches are severe and are accompanied by a rash or nausea, it could also be that you are having an allergic reaction. Prompt medical attention should be sought.

## Headaches with Fever

A headache can be expected with an infection such as flu and can usually be eased by a couple of aspirins or paracetamols. Seek help if:

  the pain is severe and the onset sudden
  there is vomiting
  neck stiffness
  a rash
  aversion to light
  high-pitched crying (children).

These symptoms appear in meningitis.

## Headaches with Fever, Facial Pain, Earache or Sore Throat

Always seek medical help, especially in children. An antibiotic may be indicated.

## Severe Pain in the Temple

Severe pain with swollen blood vessels in the temple region, sometimes with generalized muscle and joint pains: these symptoms appear in a condition called temporal arteritis (inflammation of the temporal arteries). This is a serious condition which needs urgent medical help. The middle-aged and elderly are most at risk of developing this but it is occasionally seen in younger people.

## Headaches with Eye Pain or Visual Disturbances

Report all headaches with eye pain or visual disturbances to a doctor immediately. They do occur in migraine but can also be glaucoma, a serious disease of the eye which needs prompt treatment. The symptoms come from impaired drainage of the fluid from the eye. The pain can be severe or mild and is felt around one or both eyes, or in the forehead. Nausea and vomiting may be present. Many individuals suffering from glaucoma see coloured halos around lighted objects or experience mistiness of vision. Some drugs worsen this condition, including: antihistamines, some bowel relaxants, certain tranquillizers, the tricyclic antidepressants, some anti-sickness drugs, some drugs used in Parkinson's disease.[1] Over-the-counter headache preparations should be avoided until you have seen your doctor.

While some symptoms have been highlighted in this chapter to alert you to medical emergencies, absence of these symptoms does not mean you do not need medical help. Always consult your doctor if you have headaches.

## IS IT A TUMOUR?

This is the major anxiety of most new headache sufferers. Ninety-five per cent of the population have headaches at some time. Tumours as a cause of these are rare. Other symptoms of a tumour are likely to take you to the doctor before a headache does.[2]

REFERENCES

1. Saper, Joel R., and Magee, Kenneth R., *Freedom from Headaches*, Consumers Union of United States Inc., Mount Vernon, New York, 1978
2. Blau, J. N., *Understanding Headaches and Migraine*, Which? Books, 1991

**4**

---

# The First Line of
# Investigation – the Body

## THE HEAD

You might be tempted to bypass this chapter to get to more interesting information on symptoms and what to do about them. But this would be unwise, because the more you understand the physiology of the head the easier it will be to pinpoint how you are triggering your headaches. For example, when you see how bones pulled out of alignment in the neck and shoulders can affect the circulation to the head, you will be better equipped to understand how headaches can be caused.

### The Headbone is Connected to the Neckbone

The *frontal bone* is a large flat bone forming the forehead and the roofs of the orbits where the eyes rest. It contains two cavities called the *frontal sinuses*, which lie one over each orbit towards the middle. They contain air, which enters by a small opening leading from the nose. (Remember this if you suffer from sinus problems.) These sinuses give lightness to the bone and resonance to the voice, acting as a sounding chamber. It is common for them to become infected after a cold.

The *parietal bones* are two large flat bones forming the vault of the skull (cranium). As with all bones, on their inner surface are

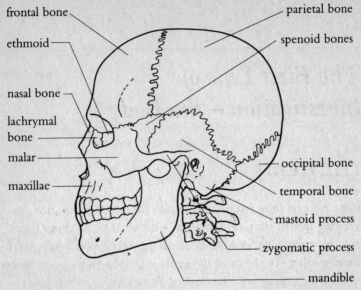

frontal bone

ethmoid

nasal bone

lachrymal bone

malar

maxillae

parietal bone

spenoid bones

occipital bone

temporal bone

mastoid process

zygomatic process

mandible

1. The bones of the head and neck

small grooves to carry the blood supply to the brain. (Remember this if you suffer tension headaches.)

The *occipital bone* is a flat bone, part of the back and base of the skull. The ridge at the base of this bone is the *occiput*. (You will be feeling for this when you use acupressure – pressure on certain points which releases tension and helps energy flow – for your headaches.) In it is a large opening, known as the *foramen magnum*, for the passage of the spinal cord. On either side of this are two pieces of bone which join with the first *vertebra*, the *atlas*, and form the joint by which the head nods. (There is information on p. 117 on the troubles caused by this bone being out of alignment.)

The *temporal bones* form the temples and also project into the base of the skull.

The *mastoid* portion goes behind the ear. A powerful muscle is attached to this. (This point can be extremely tender if you are tense.)

The *zygomatic* portion juts forward in front of the ear and joins the cheek-bone, another area where there is often pain on pressure.

The *ethmoid bone* forms the roof of the nose.

The *sphenoid bone* (shaped like a bat, after which it is named), lies in the centre of the base of the skull, joining with the frontal and ethmoid bones in front and the occipital and temporal bones at the back and on each side. Its body is in the centre of the base of the skull and has a depression on its upper surface. This houses the small but important pituitary gland and the *sphenoidal sinuses* which communicate with the nose. (Those with sinus problems please note this — sinuses are not only in the facial bones.)

The joints of the head are said to be immobile (a cranial osteopath is unlikely to agree with this), with the exception of the *temporo-mandibular joint* between the lower jaw and the skull. (More about this joint and its role in headaches in Chapter 9.) It is a loose hinge joint, so movement can take place in three ways — upwards and downwards, backwards and forwards, and from side to side. (There is a test to see if this joint is working properly on p. 119.)

Bones support the muscles, so it follows that if they are out of alignment through bad posture, repetitive movements or injury, it is unlikely that the muscles will have their full range of movement.

## Blood Supply

If you understand the position of the main blood vessels to the head you will be less likely to impede blood flow through holding your body in unnatural positions for lengthy periods. The head is supplied with food and oxygen by the *carotid arteries*, which serve the outer parts of the face and scalp, while an internal branch supplies the brain and eye.

The *vertebral arteries* run up the neck and enter an opening in the skull (foramen magnum) to supply the brain. Tight neck and shoulder muscles inhibit the blood flow to the head. The effect is similar to that caused by standing on a hosepipe when you are trying to water the garden.

## The Nerves Involved in Head Pain

The fifth cranial or *trigeminal nerve* is the major sensory nerve carrying feeling information from most of the face and scalp and also the feelings from the front portion of the tissues which cover the brain, the *meninges*. This is the nerve involved in the extreme facial pain of trigeminal neuralgia. The neck or *cervical nerves* are also important causes of head pain, since they carry sensation from the neck and the back of the head into the spinal cord and from there to the brain. This explains the phenomenon of referred pain, a pain which originates in one area and may be felt as pain in another. Pain from a dental problem can be felt in the forehead or eye, and from the neck as pain in the top or back of the head or behind the ear.

## The Brain and Electricity

The complex mechanisms of the workings of the brain are not fully understood, but it is established that, in part, it runs on electricity. Electrical currents travel from cell to cell within the brain and up and down the brain stem, spinal cord and nerves. These electrical currents are generated by the action of chemical substances, called neurotransmitters, on the cells.

Although there are many types of neurotransmitters, those which are of most importance to the headache sufferer are

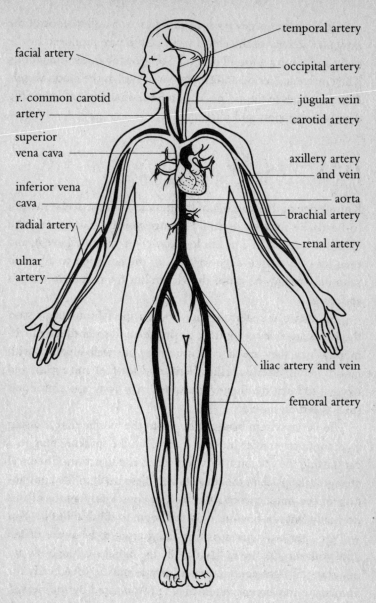

facial artery

temporal artery

occipital artery

r. common carotid artery

jugular vein

carotid artery

superior vena cava

axillery artery and vein

inferior vena cava

aorta

brachial artery

radial artery

renal artery

ulnar artery

iliac artery and vein

femoral artery

2. The circulatory system showing the main arteries and veins

*amines*. They are necessary for brain function and to control the muscular activity of the blood vessels. Some are produced by the body and some are found in food. See p. 69 for amine-rich foods. They influence mood and behaviour as well as the blood vessels. Abnormalities of the amines can cause several illnesses, including depression, anxiety and migraine.

# MUSCLES

Knowledge of the working of the muscles is of particular interest to headache sufferers: it could change you from a person who dreads the arrival of a headache, who takes pills to relieve it, and then lives on a knife-edge waiting for the next one, to a person who understands he is not the victim but the perpetrator of his suffering.

The muscular system is built up of a special muscular tissue: the fibres are able to contract or shorten and so produce movement. Since they are active tissue they are well supplied with blood vessels; arteries bring them food for fuel and repair, and oxygen to burn the fuel, while veins carry away waste products such as carbon dioxide.

The nerve system brings stimulus to the muscle fibre, causing it to contract – rather like the spark from the sparking plug in a car starting the combustion which gives rise to action. Chemical changes take place in the muscles and these result in the contraction of the muscle fibres. We are not consciously aware of this normally, but it is obvious once we begin to think about it. (You will see later how vital it is to train yourself to be aware of the state your muscles are in.) Normally the muscles of the body are in a state of slight contraction, known as muscle tone, ready for immediate movement when they are stimulated by the nerves. For example, if you see a shark swimming towards you, fear will

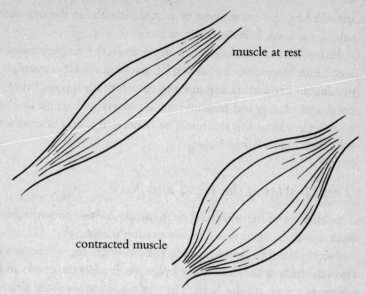

muscle at rest

contracted muscle

3. The difference between contracted and relaxed muscles

stimulate your nervous system and so your muscles will shorten to give you the extra energy needed to swim at speed for the shore.

Understanding how a continual background anxiety, even where there is no immediate threat to life or limb, can keep muscles in a state of permanent contraction could be the first step in your headache cure. During sleep and deep relaxation muscle tone is at a minimum. If a muscle is in a contracted state, overstimulated by worry, fatigue, cold or trauma, it needs to be told by the nerve impulses to relax (lengthen). The availability of its food supply and the efficiency of its waste disposal system depend on its getting the correct information.

Muscles produce action by contraction. When the contraction occurs the muscle becomes shorter, thicker and harder. When the contraction eases, the muscle becomes soft but does not automatically lengthen to its resting shape. It needs to be stretched by the contraction of another muscle on the opposite side of the joint. Muscles work in pairs.

In fact, muscles seldom work alone. Even the simplest movement usually involves the action of many muscles: for example, picking up a cup of tea requires movements of the fingers, thumb, wrist and elbow, and possibly the shoulders and trunk as the body leans forward to reach it. The concerted action of muscles is known as *muscle coordination*.

## The Muscles of the Head and Neck

The muscles of the head and neck can be divided according to their function – expression or mastication (chewing).

Notice that the *occipito-frontalis* runs over the top of the head from the back of the skull to the eyebrows. It raises the brows and moves the scalp on the head. The 'tight band around the head' headache should be less of a mystery if you imagine this muscle contracted – the effect is rather like wearing a rubber bathing cap several sizes too small. If you make a chewing movement, you will feel the muscles involved: in front of the ear (the *masseter*), in the temple (the *temporal*) and over the upper and lower jaw (the *pterygoids*). If you chew exclusively on one side there can be slight movement of the facial bones, which can lead to facial and head pain.

### Neck Muscles and Chronic Headaches

The importance of the neck muscles cannot be overemphasized. The chief muscles of the neck are the *sterno-mastoid* and the *trapezius*. The sterno-mastoid stretches from the breastbone and collar-bone and goes right up to behind the ear. Singly these muscles turn the head from side to side; used together they flex the neck. When these muscles are chronically shortened the result is pain in the head, neck and shoulders; the breath-

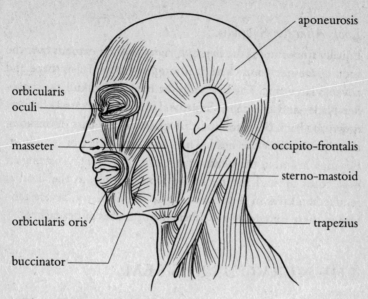

4. The muscles of the head and neck

ing can be affected, and the resulting tension can be transferred the length of the spine and even down to the knees to produce 'wobbly legs'. It is vital to keep these muscles soft and flexible.

## How Tension Affects the Head and Neck

It is only too easy to abuse these muscles by hunching your shoulders in a worried state. One reaction to tension is to hunch the shoulders and push the chin forward, rather like a short-sighted turtle peering out of its shell. Spending long periods on the telephone inclining the head to one side, viewing a badly placed television set or turning your head while working at a VDU screen are other situations in which the head and neck muscles are overburdened.

## Look After the Shoulders!

Equally important is the *trapezius muscle*, which extends over the back of the neck and chest. It is roughly triangular in shape and covers a large area. The base joins the base of the skull, the shoulder-blades and the collar-bone, and the point extends halfway down the back. So it follows that spasm in any part of this long muscle can affect the head. The combined effect of tension in this muscle and in the sterno-mastoid is equivalent to placing an iron collar around the neck: the blood supply to the head is reduced and this in turn alters the brain chemistry. Severe tension in these muscles is one of the major causes of headaches.

# THE NERVOUS SYSTEM

The nervous system controls all the functions of the body. If you ignore signals from your nervous system telling you to slow down you are in the front line for headaches. It makes sense to understand a little about how it works.

## How It Communicates

Various parts of the body communicate by a network rather like a telephone exchange. The brain is the central switchboard, the spine is the main cable and the nerves are the telephone lines which carry the messages. It consists of the central nervous system and the autonomic nervous system.

## The Central Nervous System

This is in charge of voluntary movement and is responsible for all sensations in muscles, bones and joints. It is under the control of the will – you desire to pick up a fork, so you reach out your hand and do so. This system is efficient unless it is neurologically impaired or, in times of terror, when you are paralysed with fear.

## The Autonomic Nervous System

This controls all involuntary muscles (not under the control of the will), such as internal organs, blood vessels and so on. This system is under the control of the emotions; for example, anger will cause your blood pressure to rise, fear will make the stomach churn. It has two parts: the *sympathetic*, which has a stimulating effect and the *parasympathetic*, which has a calming effect.

Think of the *sympathetic nervous system* as the man on a Harley Davidson speeding along with his foot hard down on the accelerator pedal; think of the *parasympathetic nervous system* as the man ambling around in walking boots looking at the scenery.

All the internal organs have two sets of nerves, one stimulating, the other quietening.

# Red Alert! The Action of the Sympathetic Nervous System

Imagine an air/sea-rescue helicopter crew who have had a cry for help. Their nervous systems are 'sympathetic' to their emotions and prepare their bodies to fight for their own survival and also to bring the crew of a small boat to safety.

## How Does the Nervous System Do This?

By reacting to the men tightening their muscles, which in turn squeeze their glands (rather like squeezing oranges), which then produce 'juice' – the chemical called *adrenalin*. As a result, their blood pressure rises, their heart rate speeds up, they breathe more rapidly (they need more oxygen because of the increased effort) and they sweat profusely to keep cool. To further help their efforts, blood is diverted from the abdomen to the legs so that they have more energy to move quickly. This is the reason for that sinking feeling in the tummy when we are afraid. With a reduced blood supply to the digestive organs when we are ready for action, we do not think of food or of the need to go to the lavatory. When the sympathetic nervous system is in action the adrenalin/anxiety levels are high.

## How Does the Body Revert to Normal Adrenalin Levels?

Red alert was triggered by the helicopter crew tightening their muscles, so when the all-clear is sounded, they relax their muscles. When all the survivors are safely tucked up in the ambulance, the crew relax and different chemicals are released to give the opposite effect to adrenalin. This is the parasympathetic system working efficiently; the blood pressure drops, the heart rate and breathing slow down, the sweating ceases, the blood comes back into the abdomen from arms and legs – the crewmen realize they are ready for a pie and a pint of beer, and they also make haste for the lavatory. They feel relaxed, their muscles are comfortable. The skin becomes warmer, the levels of lactic acid and cortisone in the bloodstream fall, there is an increase in the electrical resistance of the skin and the brain's wave patterns change to slow alpha waves. The adrenalin/anxiety levels are low.

# Over-stimulated Nerves Cause Headaches

It is easy to see from this why the nerves get exhausted when people have repeated stresses, conscious and unconscious (even minor ones). They keep us in a state of red alert all the time. It is equivalent to the rescue team going back and forth to the boat long after the last survivor is safe. They want to switch off the red alert but can't. Their adrenalin (and therefore anxiety) levels are still too high.

## *The Inability to Switch Off*

You might have experienced this when you have been so wound up that you carried on working long after you needed to, even though you were exhausted.

The nervous system affects all systems in the body, the glands, the circulation, the muscles, the breathing and the internal organs, so it is worth looking to its needs.

# THE RESPIRATORY SYSTEM

You might think that breathing is automatic and therefore does not need much attention. This is far from the case, for while we do not need to breathe consciously, we can develop poor breathing

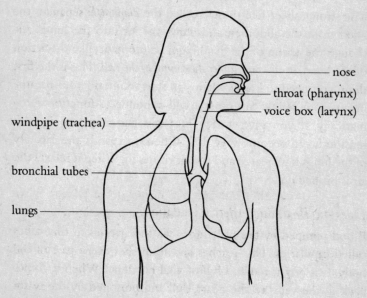

5. The respiratory system

habits which upset the nervous system and trigger, not only headaches, but also a multitude of other problems. These are discussed in Chapter 12. The respiration system consists of the lungs – two spongy sacs – and the air passages leading to them. The air passages are the nose, the *throat* (pharynx), the *voice box* (larynx), the *windpipe* (trachea) and the *bronchial tubes*.

## How the Air is Circulated

When we breathe in through the nose air is warmed and germs and other impurities are filtered out. When we breathe in through the mouth this does not happen. The result is a parched tongue, dry throat and often a cough. You must have noticed this when you have a blocked nose. This will also be familiar to those with sinus or allergy headaches.

## The Diaphragm

The strong, sheet-like muscle called the *diaphragm* separates the chest from the abdomen and draws the air into the lungs. Although the action of the diaphragm is automatic, like the action of the heart, it *can come under the control of the will*. This is the first thing you need to know when you start to retrain your breathing (p. 166). While this muscle will continue to function automatically, if you give it lazy messages and imprison it with tension it can become very dull. When it expands, the capacity of the lungs is increased and the air rushes in. When it relaxes the air is pushed out.

## Does the Breathing Affect Circulation?

Blood pumped by the heart goes via the arteries to tiny tubes called capillaries. This reaches and nourishes every part of the body. It is bright red and full of vital nutrients. When it comes back in the veins to the heart, dull and poisoned by the waste products of metabolism (the process of burning the food we eat), it goes to the lungs, where a clean-up operation is started. The success of that operation depends on how you breathe.

When you read the chapter on hyperventilation, look back to Figure 5. It will make more sense when you realize that chronic low-grade hyperventilators use only the top part of the lungs.

# DIGESTION

Although it would seem to be unrelated to the head, a faulty digestive system can be responsible for several types of headaches. Incomplete digestion due to lack of *enzymes* (the chemicals necessary to break down food), an imbalance of the good and bad bacteria in the bowel, excess fermentation, or constipation can all contribute to chronic headaches. An unhealthy bowel is unable to manufacture some of the vitamins necessary for optimum health and can also allow undigested proteins to escape into the bloodstream, causing the headaches of food intolerance (more about this on pp. 112 ff.).

## The Mouth
If meals are rushed, the important first stage of digestion is incomplete. When food is properly chewed it is mixed with saliva, which contains water, salts and the enzyme ptyalin, which breaks down starch. Mucus is also secreted in the mouth to lubricate the food.

## The Gullet and Stomach
The food then passes down the gullet or oesophagus to the stomach, where the contents are churned with gastric juices to be broken down, to kill germs which have been ingested and to prepare it to enter the small intestine.

31

## The Small Intestine

The functions of this coiled muscular tube, about 20–24 ft (6–7 m) in length, are digestion and absorption. Very little food is absorbed from the stomach; absorption takes place almost entirely from hair-like projections called villi on the wall of the intestines.

## The Bowel

Partially digested food then travels to a wider tube about 5–6 ft (1½–2 m) long, the bowel or colon. By the time the material reaches here there is very little food left in it. The residue consists of water, salts, cellulose (the indigestible parts of fruit and vegetables) and bacteria. Although the stomach juices have killed off most of the germs, the ideal conditions of food and moisture enable the remaining ones to join forces with those which are at home in the bowel. In the bowel water and salts are quickly absorbed, which leaves a paste called the stool or faeces. The few inches of tube which holds the stool before it is expelled is called the *rectum*. This is normally empty, but when it is full the sensation produced brings the desire to empty the bowel. This sensation frequently occurs when food or drink are taken, particularly after the first hot drink in the morning.

# THE LIVER

There are several ways that underfunctioning of the liver can cause headaches. It is the largest gland in the body and lies beneath the diaphragm on the right side of the abdomen. It produces bile, which helps to digest fat, stimulate *peristalsis* (the muscular action of the walls of the bowel) and rid the body of toxic substances such as alcohol and drugs. The liver converts excess amino acid from digested protein in body fuel and stores excess sugar as glycogen. The importance of this will be seen in Chapter 10 on low-blood-sugar headaches. It also stores the anti-anaemic factor (anaemia is a cause of headaches) and manufactures antibodies to protect the body against disease.

## THE PANCREAS

This gland lies behind the stomach and excretes *pancreatic juice*, which plays an important part in the process of digestion in the small intestine, and *insulin*, which controls the metabolism (conversion into energy) of carbohydrates (sugars). How overproduction of this can seriously affect brain chemistry and give rise to hypoglycaemic or low-blood-sugar headaches is explained in Chapter 10.

## THE LYMPHATIC SYSTEM

The lymphatic system is an important part of the immune system. It is a network of vessels all over the body. While blood circulates only through the blood vessels, lymph fluid (the straw-coloured fluid you might have seen when you have had a cut finger) circulates through the tissues themselves; it carries food, oxygen and water from the bloodstream to each individual cell and carries away the waste products. This is an important point to remember, because unlike the circulatory system the lymphatic system does not have a pump to propel it on its journey around the body and needs *movement* in the muscles (see the importance of exercise for headache sufferers, pp. 178–9) to prevent the tissues becoming waterlogged. When excess fluid collects in tissues the brain tissue can also become swollen with fluid

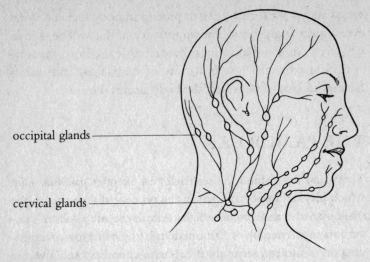

occipital glands

cervical glands

6. The lymphatic system of the head and neck

(*cerebral oedema*) and can give rise to a feeling of pressure and pain in the head.

The *lymphatic glands* are small bodies varying in size from a pea to a bean. Their function is to filter the lymph of germs as it passes through. Thus when the tissues are germ-infested the gland may become swollen and tender. If the gland has more work than it can cope with an abscess might develop. The gland also produces fresh white corpuscles for the circulation. The diagram shows the distribution of these glands in the head and neck. They are also in the abdomen. Lymphatic vessels in the abdominal organs assist in the absorption of digested food.

The lymphatic system, when working well, is an efficient garbage-disposal system. After filtration by the glands the lymph is emptied back into the circulatory system, from which the fluid in the tissues is constantly renewed.

# 5

## *Muscular-contraction or Tension Headaches*

Tension or muscular-contraction headaches probably affect more people than any other type of headache. The word tension describes the state of the muscle. It can be tensed, or contracted, as the result of a physical or emotional trigger.

The skull rests on the vertebra and, like other bones, the vertebra (spine) and neck are held in position by tendons, ligaments and many layers of muscle. These muscles and most other muscles in the body are part of a complex system of fully automatic reflexes that help to protect us against injury. For example, if you fracture your leg the muscles contract around the break and form a 'splint' to prevent movement and further injury. Often the pain from this splint is worse than the pain from the injury itself. Another example is the tightening of the abdominal muscles (this is called guarding) to protect internal organs when the appendix becomes inflamed.

In the same way, the contracted muscles which produce your headache, rather than a punishment, are an automatic protective measure which is really saying 'Don't abuse me'.

## Emotional Triggers

Emotional triggers which cause muscles in the head and neck to react are blushing when you are embarrassed and turning pale when you are afraid. You might ask why the muscles respond with pain when the trigger is emotional distress. The answer is that the muscles of the head and neck (and indeed other muscles) cannot differentiate between emotional and physical strain, so a bone out of alignment, a strained posture, fear, a bad marriage, overwork, depression or a large gas bill could all prompt the protective 'splinting' reaction. Perhaps if we were animals we would retreat into our shells or stick our heads in the sand. Instead of that we don the 'armour' of tension – a veritable iron helmet and shoulder protector.

## Physical Triggers

*Injury*: explained above

*Posture*: holding the body in strained positions: standing badly, sitting unsupported, unbalancing the head, for example

*Bedtime television watching*: the head propped forward while you peer at the screen

*Looking down while reading*: putting a strain on the neck

*Painting a ceiling*, or working in awkward situations such as under a car or the kitchen sink

*Facial mannerisms*: frowning, squinting, jaw-clenching

*Dental tension*: prolonged chewing (gum), abnormal chewing to avoid sensitive teeth, jaw problems, teeth-grinding

*Infections*: swelling

*Eye strain*: fatigue in the muscles surrounding the eye

*Spectacle problems*: pulling the head back to look through half-glasses or bifocals

## Neck Problems and Headaches

Muscle-contraction headaches can accompany arthritis of the neck (cervical spondylitis). Patients often say their pain is due to this condition in a resigned way that suggests they are doomed to headaches for the rest of their life. This is not necessarily the case. It puzzles me that this diagnosis is so often made without any physical examination or X-ray. Is it perhaps that in persons over forty-five wear and tear in the neck joints is sometimes assumed when it is not actually present? It would seem difficult to differentiate in the absence of a history of arthritis and at least a physical examination, between cervical spondylitis and muscle spasm in the neck muscles from an emotional or physical trigger.

## Arthritis

Arthritis is an inflammation of the joints. Any joint in the body can be affected. There are several types but the most common ones are osteoarthritis and rheumatoid arthritis. Osteoarthritis is by far the most common and the incidence increases with age – wear-and-tear arthritis. Rheumatoid arthritis can develop in young people and is by far the more serious condition. It can cause severe pain and deformity leading to disability.

When there is osteoarthritis in the neck there is an increased likelihood of developing muscle-contraction headaches. This could be another 'splinting' reaction and also a response to the pain. Portions of the damaged bone can press on nerves and pinch them. The nerves react with compression, irritation and eventually inflammation. This can also happen with a slipped disc. The shock absorber or cushion between the vertebra presses on the nerve, causing pain. Both osteoarthritis and a slipped disc can cause neurological symptoms such as numbness, weakness and tingling. When the cervical spine is involved this will be felt in the arms. As has been said, a person who has a painful physical focus is also more likely to be affected by emotional triggers — fear of the pain, low mood, frustration. This adds to the tension in the neck and thus causes more headaches.

## Combination Headaches

The headaches of the chronic sufferer may have both muscular and vascular (blood-vessel) components. Superimposed on their tension headaches they can suffer periodic migraine headaches. It can also happen the other way around; migraine sufferers can get 'ordinary tension headaches'. This mechanism is easier to understand, since the migraine sufferer can induce tension in the neck muscles through fear of moving the head. Injuries to the neck such as whiplash and congenital cervical spine problems are also causes of tension headaches.

## Headaches Caused by Movement and Posture

### The Exertional Headache

This headache may have a sharp or stabbing quality and may last minutes or hours. People who are prone to headaches often suffer from this type. Physical exercise, lifting, stooping or even coughing, sneezing or yawning (which can also be a sign of low blood sugar or air hunger) can bring it on. Perhaps the headache associated with lovemaking also comes into this category.

### Orgasmic Headache

These are thought to be caused by an increase in blood pressure, which causes the blood vessels in the head to dilate. The pain can be intense and may appear just before or during orgasm. It can last for minutes or several hours. The following may help:

- two aspirin or paracetamol tablets before intercourse
- a cool shower or pack to the back of the neck before intercourse
- keeping as cool as possible during lovemaking
- keeping the head as elevated as possible during lovemaking
- a strong cup of coffee before intercourse could constrict the blood flow to the head.

### Hairdressing Headache

Some people get a dull headache after a visit to the hairdresser's, where they have held their head back over the basin for a shampoo. The headache arrives later in the day or the following morning. It can be avoided by bending forward over the basin.

## What Happens When the Muscles in the Head or Neck are Tense?

A mechanical failure develops which produces brain symptoms and local symptoms. The blood vessels constrict, the brain chemistry is altered because it can't function properly without an adequate blood flow, and pain and stiffness develop in the muscles (the fibres contract) because they are not being adequately nourished either; another reason for the pain is a build-up of the waste products of metabolism in the tissues.

## Stopping the Washing-machine Mid-cycle

You will remember that a healthy lymphatic system takes nourishment to the cells and then carries the garbage away. When the muscles are contracted the waste products are trapped in the tissues and crystalline deposits form in the muscles in the same way that soap deposits would collect in your shirt if you repeatedly washed it and turned the dial to Spin Dry before it had been through the rinsing cycle. These deposits are another source of pain, although the sufferer, because of restricted movement, may not realize just how much trouble the garbage in the muscles is causing until a downward pressure is exerted on the muscles covering the shoulder-blades. This is often very painful and if the condition becomes chronic the tissues can become inflamed and swollen.

In muscular-contraction headaches the blood vessels are usually constricted, but like any other muscular tube under strain periodic striving to correct the position can cause dilation which would be felt as sharp stabs of pain just as in intestinal colic.

# FEATURES OF A TENSION HEADACHE

## Distribution of Pain

The pain is usually dull on the top of the head, extending from the forehead like a tight band and can go down the back of the head, behind the ear, into the jaw and across the face. The muscles at the base of the skull are often very tender on pressure. The pain can extend further, to the neck, shoulders and upper back.

## When Does the Pain Start?

It can come at any time of the day but rarely starts in the night. It usually affects both sides and can produce a feeling of a weight on the top of the head or a tight band around the head accompanied by a 'spacy' feeling. Sufferers can go to bed with a headache and wake up with the same headache. This is more common in people who are anxious and depressed. Their subconscious works away all night trying to help resolve their emotional conflicts and the result is that they awake as tense as when they retired to bed. It is more usual, however, for the pain to start in the morning and gradually worsen as the day progresses, with sleep bringing some measure of relief.

## How Long Does the Headache Last?

It can last hours, days or even weeks if nothing is done about it. It is easy to understand why these headaches can be protracted. When the muscles are habitually overstimulated they become so contracted that merely switching off by reading, watching television or sleeping is not enough to allow them to rest in their lengthened state. The muscles need practical help in the form of stretching, massage, acupressure or other hands-on treatment, or the person might resort to painkillers, muscle relaxants or alcohol. The drawbacks of using drugs and alcohol are discussed later.

## Who Suffers from This Type of Headache?

Both sexes (in about equal proportions) and all ages. They usually start in early adult life although 10–20 per cent of sufferers have their first attacks in childhood.[1]

## Children and Tension

One might imagine that children would escape tension in the head, neck and shoulders, because they are supple and active and don't have the responsibilities of adult life. This is definitely not so; life is different but just as difficult for them. The neuroses of later life are incubated during the early years. Children often find it difficult to express emotional pain and this can be missed by the adults around them. It is impossible to have all our needs met even if we are born into loving, stable families – the world is a fearful place. We react to this fear by tightening our muscles or 'armouring'. This practical mechanism allows us to hold in our fear, frustration, anger, grief, sadness or any other hurtful emotion. Thus the foundation stone of neurosis is laid. For more about this see Shirley Trickett, *Coping with Anxiety and Depression* (Sheldon, 1989).

In children, physical triggers causing muscle tension include the persistent cough which keeps the shoulders raised, badly placed desks and pushing the head forward to peer at the blackboard. Sleeping on the stomach can put a strain on the neck, as can being carried on the mother's hip and having to turn the head in one direction to see the world. Sadly, also, children often spend long hours in front of badly positioned TV sets or lying on the floor lifting the head up to play computer games.

## Appearance of a Person with a Tension Headache

They are usually very pale, because of the constriction of the blood vessels, the face lacks expression and the eyes look dull. The sufferer often looks detached, as though they are not quite with you. If there are sinus problems in addition to the tension headache there can be dull red patches over the cheek-bones and fluid retention around the eyes. Sometimes the face can look puffy. This is probably because of congestion due to the tight muscles impeding the lymph drainage from the head. Furrowing of the brow can also be a feature.

# Symptoms Which Can Accompany the Headache

- Visual disturbances: these are not as dramatic as in migraine sufferers, but they can occur in tension headaches, usually in the form of blurred vision or, if it is severe, there can be altered perception. In a *hallucination* the person sees something that is not there – for example a pink elephant. In *altered perception* the person sees what is there – for example, a flower on a curtain may appear like a face.

- Pain in the neck, shoulders and back.
- Bloating of the stomach or bowel and wind. Often the passing of wind is the first sign that the headache is abating. Nausea and loss of appetite are often part of the symptom picture, or craving for foods not normally a part of the sufferer's diet.
- Shakiness and lack of muscular coordination: for example, difficulty gripping a pen or clumsiness and regularly dropping things.
- Fatigue and lack of interest in things normally enjoyed.
- Wobbly legs: feelings of not quite knowing where the ground is or of walking on eggshells.
- Dizziness, especially when turning the head.
- Irritability, anxiety, depression and feeling of unreality; for example, walking into the kitchen and it being unfamiliar; or depersonalization – when a person looks into the mirror and they know intellectually it is their image they see but somehow they look different, rather like a distorted image in a mirror at a funfair.
- Difficulty in breathing through the nose – mild hyperventilation.

Some of these symptoms might seem rather remote from the site of pain, but because they happen with such monotonous regularity, most people are very accurate about their symptom picture; and the same symptoms crop up again and again in large numbers of people.

The pain is less disabling than migraine. Most sufferers continue working through these headaches and rarely retreat to bed during the day. Many people accept their headaches almost as a way of life.

# ARE YOUR MUSCLES TENSE?

1. Tilt your head back and gaze at the ceiling. If this makes you feel dizzy the muscles of your neck could be part of your problem.
2. (Not for those with back problems.) Standing up and keeping your knees straight, see how far you can easily reach to your toes. Do not strain. If you cannot reach much below your knees then your back muscles are tense.

# TYPICAL EXPERIENCES

## Woman of Thirty

I had been having tension headaches for almost a year before I pinpointed what they were. I could carry on working but the headaches were beginning to get me down. It was all a bit of a mystery to me. If I had been anxious or depressed perhaps it would have been easier to understand. My life was going well. I had a new job, which was exciting and hectic, I moved to a better flat and bought a car. For the first few months I was on cloud nine. Then began what I can only describe as a feeling of fullness and nausea in the muscles of my neck and shoulders. The headaches started with feelings of my head being heavy and sometimes I had an overwhelming desire to go to sleep. Over the weeks it changed to a dull continual ache in the whole of my head and the right side of my neck and my right shoulder. A couple of times I thought I was getting flu but nothing developed. I then thought it was perhaps sinus headaches and tried some nasal decongestant tablets from the chemist's. These didn't help

much so I saw my doctor. He said they were tension headaches and gave me painkillers. If I took them regularly
throughout the day they did ease the pain but I did not
like the feeling that went with them. They gave me a
muzzy head and I felt tired. I stopped taking them after a
few weeks. The headaches came back with full force and I
did not get any relief or real insight into how I was bringing them on until the computers were off at work for two
days following a weekend. During this enforced break my
head cleared considerably. I had to admit that my boyfriend was right when he argued that it was the stress at
work. I could not see this because I was thoroughly enjoying my job. I made a big effort to slow down: got up earlier
and made time to have breakfast and pack food for lunch
(there was no canteen at this job and I had been having a
doughnut or sausage roll for lunch). My boyfriend massaged my neck and shoulders with olive oil each night and
I made a neck pillow from a rolled towel bound with a
crêpe bandage. I stretched my neck regularly throughout
the day and tried not to hunch my shoulders. Making sure
I did not sit for any more than forty-five minutes at my
desk at work without having a walk around the office was
the hardest thing. I felt rather silly always wandering
around. If I work late too often or get myself uptight about
anything the pain comes back but generally it is very much
better and I feel in control now – it does not control me.
The muscles in my neck and shoulder are still very tender
and this reminds me that the headaches are still lurking in
the background and will come back if I am not vigilant.

This experience illustrates that the nervous system not only
cannot distinguish between physical and emotional triggers for
headaches but also that it does not matter whether the cause is

painful or pleasurable. The new job and exciting life caused the problem.

## Woman of Forty-three

I had never been a headachy person so I was mystified by the severe headaches which appeared out of the blue. I felt sick and shaky with them and my neck and shoulders ached and felt like a ton weight. Paracetamol took the edge off it but the relief did not last long. They were worse at the end of the day and I began to dread going to work.

After about three months I went to an osteopath to see if there was something wrong with my neck. He said the muscles were in spasm and asked me if I had been doing anything different over the months. I could not think that I had. I was in the same job and had not had any added strain. I worked as a secretary but my desk was in good light by a window. When he asked me how long it was since I had been to have my eyes tested I said it could not be anything to do with my eyes because I had bought new glasses about four months earlier. He swooped on this and asked if they were half-glasses. They were, in fact. I had chosen them because the plastic frames had been making a red mark on my nose and I thought these would be lighter. He then explained what I had been doing – pulling my head back to see the full screen of my word processor through the lens. He pulled my head into that position and my muscles felt really sore. I could not imagine how I had missed this. He adjusted the bones of my neck and I went back for a few sessions of massage with an electrical thing and the headaches have gone. I went back to my old glasses until I got some fibreglass full-framed ones. My vanity over a red mark on my nose had caused months of headaches!

## Man of Forty-seven

My job entails hours of driving and I had blamed the fumes of the traffic and irregular hours for my persistent headaches. I had been to the doctor to have my blood pressure checked. He said I was a bit overweight but everything else seemed fine and advised me to cut down on drinking and take more exercise. I was a regular drinker but not vast quantities. I did this and started walking more but there was no improvement. I had my eyes tested and they were unchanged since the last visit.

If it had not been for the back pain I would probably still be having the headaches. I turned to open the fridge and my back went. It was excruciating. The doctor seemed unconcerned. He told me to lie flat for a few days and gave me muscle relaxants. I had never had back pain before and was convinced that there was something very seriously wrong. Within a week I felt much better and went back to work. On my first long drive my head throbbed and I was aching all down my back. My neck felt barely able to support my head.

It was my wife's lack of sympathy that finally made me do something. She said living with me was miserable and although she did not actually voice it I felt she was hinting that she would leave me. She had left me briefly years before. She insisted I went to a stress management course.

The first evening was a waste of time but the second was on stress caused by driving. This did make sense. The instructor showed what happened when the head was pushed forward for long hours to peer at the road. I realized that I had been doing this and that my seat was not right. I bought a back support (I am not very tall) and put a cushion in the small of my back. I could feel the difference almost at once. I have also become more aware of how I move and how I sit when relaxing. I began to eat more fruit and vegetables and lost half a stone in weight. I still get the odd headache but they are nothing like what they were.

This account highlights the fact that keeping the head in an unbalanced position for protracted periods throws the whole spine out of alignment – the tension goes to the neck and shoulders, and then travels down the back.

## Woman of Sixty

I had put up with headaches for years and if I had not developed panic attacks I might still be having them. The headaches I had coped with, but the panic attacks sent me rushing to the doctor. They were so terrifying, I did not think of them as panic attacks. I felt as though I was dying or at least had some very serious illness. The doctor tried to reassure me but I was not convinced. He said that they were just a sign that I had been under stress. That was what I could not understand because it was the first time for years that I was *not* under stress – my time was my own since my invalid mother had gone to live with my sister. I was really happy about her being there and was enjoying reading and gardening and, best of all, a full night's sleep. It was all very puzzling. I searched the bookshops for information on panic attacks and had to admit that the doctor must have been right – the feelings I was getting, palpitations, sweating, feeling unable to breathe and desperate feelings of fear and feeling that something dreadful was going to happen were all there. It said they were more common in people who had symptoms of tension such as headaches and neck aches. I had thought that perhaps the headaches were due to an old whiplash injury. I had never felt particularly tense and I certainly did not feel unhappy.

The headaches and panic attacks persisted and it was not until I was afraid to go out that the doctor arranged for a community psychiatric nurse to come to see me. It was her explanation which finally convinced me I was not dying of something terrible. She explained that after years of strenuous activity looking after Mother, suddenly my body had no need of the adrenalin which had kept me going and that my body was still producing so much that it flooded over the top causing panic attacks. She taught me how to calm down, breathe slowly and let my muscles relax. She also accompanied me on shopping trips until I could go out alone. I don't get headaches now and the panic attacks have decreased to just an odd flutter in the stomach now and then.

This experience is an example of how after years of pressing the panic button to produce lots of adrenalin, the body is not able to adjust overnight to you saying that it is time to relax – the panic is over.

## Woman of Thirty-four

I had suffered headaches since I was about four years old. My mother did not take much notice of them – she just gave me junior aspirin and told me to lie down or go out in the fresh air. I had the feeling that she did not really believe me, and as I got older I felt she thought I was inventing them to avoid school or duck some chore I did not want to do. This was probably the case sometimes but I know I did not imagine the headaches because they also often prevented me doing things I wanted to do. I can still remember the weight at the back of my neck and the feeling that my arms would not move properly. The headaches also made my eyes hurt and sometimes I felt sick. Looking back I can see I was a loving child, very anxious to please, lonely and frightened. My parents rowed constantly and although I never saw any violence I always worried in case they would hurt each other. I used to lie in bed when they presumably thought I was asleep and pull the covers over my head to shut out the noise of their shouting.

They were not bad parents and I'm sure they loved me, and still do, in their way, but they seemed totally unaware of the effect their relationship had on me.

I stayed at home until I was twenty in the mistaken belief that my presence would somehow help the situation and also perhaps because I was nervous about moving away.

The headaches became worse after I left school. I did not have a job and spent a lot of time in the house.

When I finally decided to go to college (encouraged by my aunt) I moved as far away as I could. It was the best thing I ever did. My parents separated. It seemed that far from helping the situation I had kept it going. They were staying together until I left home.

The headaches completely vanished a couple of months after I left home. It was a really odd feeling, as though there was a space where the weight should have been.

I met a boy in the first week at university doing the same course. We now live together. At first I was very anxious about visiting home in the holidays but I have got over that now and I'm fine unless I have to see my parents together.

This young woman's story outlines how constant nagging fear at any age can trigger headaches – a purely emotional cause in an otherwise healthy person. Whatever the cause the physiological end result is the same.

## Man of Fifty-two

I started having headaches a couple of weeks after I was made redundant. I think I was in a state of shock. I had worked for the same firm for fourteen years, got up at the same time, met the same people every day and then suddenly it was all gone, and added to that I had the worry of how I was going to carry on paying my mortgage and supporting my family.

The pain started with a dull ache at the base of my skull which I could move with a couple of aspirins but when they got fiercer the pills did not work. They went on and on and I eventually went to the doctor. He said he could give me headache tablets but he felt the real trouble was depression and that he would rather give me antidepressants. I was very much against drugs and refused, and also refused his offer to see a counsellor. I felt I had to work it out for myself.

A month later I was glad to go back and take the antidepressants. I got up with a headache and went to bed with a headache. Things were going from bad to worse. I was very irritable and my wife was showing signs of strain.

I felt horrible for the first week on the pills. My headache was just the same and added to it I had a queer, otherworldly feeling. I was tempted to stop them but my wife encouraged me to carry on. The doctor did say it would be a few weeks before I felt the benefit. After a couple of weeks I was getting more sleep – not waking at the crack of dawn with thoughts rushing around in my head – and from then on things improved.

I have been on them eight weeks now and can't say I'm back to normal (how can I be without a job?) but things don't seem so black and my head is a great deal better. I don't intend to carry on with the pills long-term. I just need a rest to pull up and get myself motivated again. I am thinking of applying for a grant to start a small business.

This experience shows how headaches can start after a shock and can be very much part of anxiety and depression. Many people live in a permanent state of low-grade depression without even realizing what is wrong. They accept continual headaches and fatigue as a way of life and struggle on through the greyness, often fiercely denying that they are depressed. It is as though they accept the physical pain and it protects them from really looking at what is wrong in their lives. It could be an unhappy marriage or a job where they are completely unfulfilled or a situation where they continually subjugate their needs to the needs of others and underneath feel resentful and angry. Often looking at these issues and bringing them into the open is far more scary than covering them up with headaches.

## Woman of Fifty

I had suffered migraine headaches when I was a teenager but I knew the recent headaches were something different. Unfortunately I traced the cause, or rather my daughter did, to my new shoulder-bag. I loved it. It was black leather with a tan trim. It was bigger and heavier than my old one and as usual (my handbags were a family joke) it was full of rubbish. I had been complaining of headaches for a couple of weeks but it was not until I mentioned my sore shoulder that my daughter said it could be the bag. I had been having a great time at the sales and had been on several trips to town. The pain was all on the left, bag-carrying side; in my neck, shoulder, jaw and eye. I also had a tight feeling in my head and felt a bit spaced out.

I took some ibuprofen, changed my bag for my daughter's, which went around my middle, and did some stretching exercises. The headaches went after about a week and so far I have not had any more.

## Man of Thirty-seven

I had been a tension-headache sufferer for years and they were getting worse. Alexander lessons (see Chapter 18) completely cured them. It is not something I would have considered if I had not seen the improvement in my wife. Her back had been in trouble for years and she was a different person after the treatment.

The teacher showed me how I was building tension into just about every movement I made. I have to admit I found it tedious at times and rather expensive but I would certainly go back if I was ever in trouble again.

These will probably not match your experience exactly; they are simply intended to illustrate how a wide variety of emotional and physical factors (some of which seem unlikely) can trigger tension headaches. Anything which pulls your body around or is a nagging worry in your subconscious can be all that it takes.

## REFERENCES

1. Saper, Joel R., and Magee, Kenneth R. *Freedom from Headaches*, Consumers Union of United States Inc., Mount Vernon, New York 1978

# 6

## Migraine

### Common, Classical, Cluster Headaches

Ten per cent of the population of the UK suffer from migraine. The condition affects both sexes, all age groups, 'civilized' and primitive peoples. Even babies can suffer from migraine. The word is often used to describe any severe headache which no one knows how to cure. The inaccuracy of this should become apparent as you read on.

### Migraine in Literature

Many writers have described their migraine attacks in their stories. They include Shakespeare, Anthony Trollope, G. K. Chesterton and Rudyard Kipling. Perhaps the most notable is Lewis Carroll – even his images suggest the visual disturbances of a migraine attack and his text often refers to the severe pain. Tweedledum comments in *Through the Looking Glass*, ' "I'm very brave, generally," he went on in a low voice: "only today I happen to have a headache." ' Tweedledum's heavy headgear is also an indication of what the writer is feeling. ' "Do I look very pale?" said Tweedledum, coming up to have his helmet tied on. (He *called* it a helmet, though it certainly looked much more like a saucepan)' . . .

## The Migraine Attack

This could be said to be a collection of symptoms usually involving severe recurring headache, thought to be vascular (constriction usually followed by dilation of the blood vessels to the brain) in origin, in a person where full investigations fail to reveal an organic cause and where typical symptoms accompany different phases of the attack. For example, mood changes in the prodromal (warning) phase, followed by severe headache, with or without digestive symptoms such as nausea, vomiting, bloating and diarrhoea, and also neurological symptoms (in classical migraine), which include visual disturbances, paraesthesia (pins and needles), clumsiness or transient paralysis. Recovery is usually after the 'hangover' phase, in which the sufferer feels exhausted. The sequential nature of each set of symptoms plus the length of time of each phase clearly distinguishes it from other types of headaches such as muscular (tension) headaches, although it is possible for a migraine sufferer also to be prone to tension headaches, and at times they might even coexist.

The term 'migraine' is of French origin, but its root is from the Greek term *hemicrania*, meaning affliction of half of the head.

## What's in a Word?

Not a lot in this case! How can one word describe several distinct conditions which constitute the phenomenon of migraine, some of which can bring a plethora of frightening, disabling and bizarre symptoms. Any new sufferers who have been diagnosed as having migraine and who seek confirmation and reassurance from a dictionary are likely to be disappointed, particularly if they have the type of migraine which involves neurological symptoms.

## Attitudes to Migraine

Migraine attacks have been recorded historically for over two thousand years. It is astonishing that for a condition which has been around for so long and affects 10 per cent of people in the United Kingdom alone, there is limited understanding and still no medical cure. Prescribed drugs help some people to lead near-normal lives but many of them bring their own problems. What is even more unfathomable than the limited help available is the archaic attitude towards the condition. It is generally regarded just as a tiresome headache, visited upon tiresome people, who through their tiresomely regular visits to the surgery, their frequent absences from work ('she's/he's having another one of her/his migraines'), their frequent retreats to lie down in a darkened room, deliberately make life tiresome for those around them. If your pancreas fails to secrete insulin and you develop diabetes you are unlikely to encounter any problems – swift diagnosis, effective treatment, continued support. The same happens if you develop another 'respectable' condition like pernicious anaemia – injections of vitamin $B^{12}$, continued care – no hint that you are malingering. Better still if some part of you can be replaced, removed or treated with some high-tech medicine – all very respectable.

## Why is Migraine Such a Poor Relation in Medicine?

Firstly because it is non-life-threatening, and secondly because it involves changes in brain chemistry and therefore alteration in mood and behaviour. When a spanner is thrown into the works of the great neurochemical factory, the brain (about which science admits it still has a lot to learn), there is bound to be a multiplicity of symptoms. Perhaps it is these which lead non-sufferers to believe that migraine is a rather nasty headache – but everyone gets a headache at some time! – with a hint of hypochondria.

# WHAT HAPPENS DURING AN ATTACK

Migraine could be described as a disorder of arousal. Placid people are less likely to suffer but are not immune. The brain stem, the oldest part of the brain, controls the autonomic nervous system, which oversees body functions such as the muscular activity of the digestive system, breathing, circulation and sensory perceptions, sound, touch, taste, hearing and smell. It also includes the reticular activating system (RAS). This mechanism determines how much stimulation is allowed to reach the brain. For example, two people who go to the same party will have RAS systems which react differently. A has an RAS system which is partly closed but still alert enough to react if there was danger such as a fire in the building. B has an RAS system which is wide open and reacts much more to the stimuli around him. A is likely to go home and relax into a sound sleep. B is likely to be overstimulated long after leaving the noise and excitement of the party. The inability to relax might make him resort to tranquillizers or alcohol to induce sleep. A and B have both had the same stimulation but react differently.

The lymbic system is controlled by the hypothalamus, which prompts the release of chemicals from the pituitary and adrenal glands. It is unable to distinguish between the signals of fear or pain and pleasure or excitement. When the senses are not being stimulated the hypothalamus reduces the supply of stress hormones and secretes endorphins which produce a state of relaxation. The hypothalamus has a high concentration of the neurotransmitter serotonin (see p. 68), which is a chemical messenger between nerve cells.

# TAKING YOUR MIGRAINE TO THE DOCTOR

Doctors' reactions to migraine vary a great deal. A consultation can be caring and very thorough, or it can be caring but lacking in helpful information or treatment, or sadly, as is so often the case, it can be dismissive and hurtful. This may be because the doctor is irritated with the patient for making a fuss about what he sees as 'just a headache', or it can be that the practitioner is angry with himself over his own inadequacy in the management of migraine – he has nothing other than a prescription for pain-killers, which he knows are of limited use, to offer the patient.

## *Typical Experiences of a Consultation*

I was very frightened when I arrived at the surgery utterly convinced I was going to die from a brain tumour. I felt something serious must be going wrong in my head to cause such excruciating pain and to affect my vision and speech. After a detailed history, including questions about my relatives, the doctor said he was almost certain that my problem was migraine, but this could not be confirmed until I had been examined and had undergone some rou-tine tests. *Migraine!* I listened to this with a mixture of dis-belief and relief. The doctor said he was referring me to a neurologist at the Migraine Clinic, who he felt sure would confirm the diagnosis.

I left the surgery feeling better although not totally con-vinced. I was given a prescription for painkillers and a leaf-let about migraine. The leaflet aroused my fears again. It did not describe anything like I was experiencing. It was brief and mentioned more about triggers than symptoms. I felt desperate to see the symptoms I was having under the heading 'Migraine'. I think that would have convinced me.

The doctor was very kind and reassuring but I still wondered if he was holding something back from me. In retrospect I realize I was in such a state of anxiety it would have taken a lot to put my mind at ease.

I have had migraine for seven years. The need to take more and more time off work drove me to see my GP. It was a waste of time. I felt anxious and rushed as I tried to explain the symptoms, worried that I was leaving something vital out. He looked at my notes all the time and I wondered if he was listening to me.

After taking my blood pressure and looking into my eyes he said, you have had headaches a long time. There is nothing to suggest they are anything more than migraine. Would you like some painkillers? I was in and out in five minutes.

After years of unhelpful, dismissive consultations with my doctor I gave up making appointments. I always felt worse when I came out, almost as if I were to blame for the pain. It was when I had an attack at work and saw the works' doctor that I got some help. He gave me an injection to stop the vomiting and made me lie down. He asked me to make an appointment to see him the following week for a chat. I had more information in that twenty-minute conversation than I had ever had. No one had ever explained what happens during an attack and what changes I could make in my lifestyle to lessen attacks. He recommended some reading and gave me an address to send off for a relaxation tape. I walked out on air — I had previously thought of migraine as something one just 'had'—something that you just had to live with.

# TYPES OF MIGRAINE

The condition described as *common* migraine accounts for 80 per cent of migraine attacks. The rarer *classical* migraine has been recorded historically for over two thousand years and has a more complicated, well-defined symptom picture. Both types usually share the symptom of a severe headache. *Cluster* headache is rarer and can be easily distinguished from the other types.

## The Stages of a Migraine Attack

1. Warning or pre-headache phase
2. The aura (classical migraine)
3. The headache
4. The postdromal or 'hangover' phase

# COMMON MIGRAINE

## The Warning Phase

The pre-headache phase is seen in both common and classical migraine although it is not experienced by all common migraine sufferers. It may last for a few hours or even for several days before an attack. The phase may include:

mood changes
tension
irritability
confusion
mental dullness
vertigo
fainting

fatigue
weight gain
nausea
hunger
stuffy nose
raised blood pressure
extra energy
euphoria.

## The Headache Phase

The pain can last for a few hours to three days and is described by most sufferers as hot and pulsating; it affects the head, face, jaw and sometimes the neck and shoulder area. The latter may be the result of holding the head in a fixed position, since the slightest movement or coughing or sneezing can increase the pain. The pain may be worse on one side and attacks frequently occur around the time of menstruation. The sufferer usually notices the headache on waking, although it can actually wake them up.

Vomiting, diarrhoea and constipation are frequently present, and these can lead to dehydration. The sufferer often describes their affliction as 'sick headaches'. Sufferers may feel hot/cold/sweaty, but a recent study by Dr J. N. Blau and Dr E. Anne Macgregor of the City of London Migraine Clinic showed that recorded temperatures were normal. Acute sensitivity to light, sound and smell can also be present. Neurological symptoms are rare in common migraine.

## Abating of Headache

Symptoms improve with time and loss of body fluids through vomiting, diarrhoea, increased flow of urine, tears, sweating or streaming nose.

## The Hangover Phase

The sufferer often feels drained of energy and has to move slowly. Even thinking can be an effort.

# CLASSICAL MIGRAINE

## The Pre-headache Phase

Typically, classical migraine sufferers report that the aura is the first sign of an attack, but in some people the pre-headache phase is also experienced. This is sometimes called the 'prodrome', from the Greek *prodromos* meaning 'coming before'. The experience can be one of fearfulness and depression, or of feeling very well, full of energy and creativity.

## The Aura

This is thought to arise from disturbances in the blood flow to the head. The symptoms depend on which part of the brain is affected. They can be frightening and bizarre and people often think they are going mad or having a stroke. The aura may only last for fifteen to twenty minutes before the onset of the headache.

### Visual Disturbances

hypersensitivity to light
blurred vision
double vision

} these appear in both types of migraine, but are not the aura symptoms; they are noted here for convenience

partial blindness

blind spot in one or both eyes (scotoma)
tunnel vision
figures appear elongated or shortened
spots or sparkling shapes or glare

Visual disturbances often cause clumsiness and bumping into things. There can also be a distortion of body image or the sufferer may feel that part of the body is 'not there'.

## The Headache Phase

### Sensory Disturbances

acute sensitivity to slightest noise
ringing in ears
altered taste sensation
acute sensitivity to touch

### Neurological Symptoms

lack of coordination
weakness in limbs
tingling
transient paralysis
inability to grip
inability to find words
speech problems

### Organic and Circulatory Symptoms

nausea
abdominal pain
gut rumbling
belching

increased urination
thirst
diarrhoea
pseudo-angina
cold hands and feet
vertigo
fainting

### Psychological Symptoms

tension
feelings of dread
confusion
memory loss

### Visible Signs

pallor
flushing
bloodshot eyes
yawning
sweating

The headache phase can last from four to seventy-two hours in adults and less in children. The pain may initially be unilateral but as it worsens it can spread to a deep throbbing pain all over the head, behind the eyes, in the ear and jaw, and the neck and shoulders. Generalized aches and pains can also be present, plus nausea, vomiting and prostration.

## The Post-headache Phase

The person can be exhausted, confused and depressed, or sluggish, with stiff, sore muscles. Large amounts of urine can be passed and sometimes there is abnormal appetite or food cravings. Severe diarrhoea can also be a feature. A minority of people feel 'cleansed' and in high spirits. This may be due partly to relief that the attack is over, or there may be a biochemical reason similar to the sudden 'lift' some women feel after a period.

# AFTER A SEVERE MIGRAINE ATTACK

As Mary K. Henneberger points out, in a reprint from the *Newsletter* of the National Headache Foundation, Chicago, USA, the aftermath of a severe migraine is generally overlooked in headache literature and frequently ignored in treatment. Aching limbs, neck, shoulders and back may persist for several days and a deep pain or sore spot in the back, described by Oliver Sachs in *Migraine: Understanding a Common Disorder* as the post-migraine 'bruise', may be a source of discomfort for several days. Rest, the application of heat and analgesics may bring comfort.

# SOME SIMPLE MEASURES TO TRY

## The 'Pale' Phase

Initially, when the blood vessels are constricted, the following may help:

- Lie flat to increase circulation to head; raise feet on pillows.
- Apply covered hot-water bottle to back of neck or hot lavender compress to forehead (five drops of essential oil of lavender – or any oil recommended by aromatherapist or book – in a

bowl of hot water). Have two washcloths and change the cloth as soon as it cools.

• Massage scalp around the base of the skull and the neck, and gently move the shoulders.

• If well enough to stand, have a warm shower and hold the shower head close to the back of the neck.

## The 'Hot' Phase

When the blood vessels dilate the tissues become engorged with blood and swell. Try:

• Lying or sitting propped up with the head well supported to decrease circulation to head.

• Apply ice pack to nape of neck and washcloths which have been in cold water (add ice from freezer), to forehead.

• Keep the rest of the body cool.

• Get someone to massage your feet or rest them on a covered hot-water bottle.

• Apply Tiger Balm (available from health stores or Asian stores) or Oil of Olbas (widely available in pharmacists) to neck and forehead. Both of these have a cooling effect.

• Have an ionizer as near your face as possible (see p. 186).

• If you can get off the bed, have a cool shower or Epsom salts bath. This will help to remove excess water from the body. Large packs of Epsom salts are available from pharmacies. Use three cups full in warm water. Apply cool washcloth to head.

# DRUGS USED FOR MIGRAINE

This is a matter for you to discuss with your doctor and there is no doubt that for some people acute medication at times is the only effective treatment. There are, however, often unwanted side-effects and it is better to find out what is triggering your migraines rather than just treat the symptoms. Any drug taken for headaches suppresses the body's natural pain-relieving substances and if you are cutting down or cutting out medication, for a time your headaches will increase in intensity.[1] This is the analgesic rebound effect. To cut down slowly and help the body to detoxify is the only way. There is no short cut.

Before discussing some of the drugs which can induce headaches, I must stress once again that any medication you are on for any condition should not be cut down or stopped without consulting your medical practitioner.

# DRUGS WHICH CAUSE HEADACHES AND MIGRAINE

A headache is one of the first signs to indicate you have taken a substance which the body regards as a poison. To list all the drugs where headaches are a side-effect would be to reproduce half of the *British National Formulary*. Special mention could be made of one of the antidepressant drugs fluoxetine (Prozac) which, although it has been used to relieve migraine in some subjects, has also been found to produce it in a person who has never experienced a migraine attack before.[2]

## Common Drugs Which Can Cause Headaches

Some common drugs dilate the blood vessels which supply the brain and therefore produce symptoms like the engorgement phase of migraine. When they are withdrawn a rebound constriction of the blood vessels can also be a cause of headaches.

caffeine
alcohol
evening primrose oil
vitamin B3
tranquillizers and sleeping pills (benzodiazepines)
monoamine oxidase inhibitor antidepressants
nicotine

## Drugs Used for Migraine which may Produce Headaches in Non-sufferers

tricyclate antidepressants
the contraceptive pill
hormone replacement therapy
non-steroidal anti-inflammatory drugs
ergotamine

# FOOD TRIGGERS

## Amines

These are substances necessary for brain and blood-vessel function. Some are found in food, others are manufactured in the body. They serve as neurotransmitters and a disturbance in the normal balance can cause disorders such as depression, Parkinson's disease and migraine.

## Serotonin

This is an important nitrogen-containing amine and is found in a variety of tissues, including the brain. Since it constricts some blood vessels and contracts others it is not surprising that it is thought to play a key role in the production of headaches and migraine. Like other brain amines such as noradrenalin, it not only determines the size of blood vessels, but also controls mood and sleep patterns. Low levels of serotonin have been found in people who have committed suicide. High levels are known to cause mania, headaches and other problems.

The level of serotonin drops dramatically at the onset of a migraine attack, the constricted blood-vessel stage, and presumably rises rapidly with the dilation phase. Vomiting lowers serotonin levels. This could be why some people (particularly children) induce vomiting to relieve their headache. When the balance of amines is altered in the body a migraine can be triggered. When looking for the food that is triggering your migraine, remember it could be that it is the total amount of amines you are including in your diet rather than one specific food such as cheese or chocolate. Sensitivity to amine-rich foods is generally recognized by the medical profession as a trigger in migraine, although food intolerances (the leaky-gut syndrome, p. 103) as a cause of health problems is still a contentious issue in general practice.

## Amine-rich Foods

### Dairy products
Cheese – particularly mature cheeses such as Stilton, Brie and Camembert – yogurt and sour cream. There seems to be divided opinion about milk; cottage and cream cheese are generally thought not to be a problem.

### Meat
Pork, game, smoked meats, offal.

### Fish
Pickled and preserved fish.

## Yeast Extracts

Marmite, Vegemite, some stock cubes, some packet soups, miso, soy sauce, some gravy powders.

## Fruit and Vegetables

spinach
citrus fruits (particularly oranges)
bananas
figs
plums
pineapples
raisins
avocados
sauerkraut
broad beans
soya beans
onions

## Products Containing Vinegar

Pickles, relishes, salad dressings, sauces.

## Chocolate

Confectionery, chocolate desserts, chocolate drinks.

# Alcohol

All alcoholic drinks, particularly red wines, beer, sherry and some white wines. The effects of alcohol can be twofold: dilating the blood vessels and raising the amine levels. You can also be allergic to the corn in whisky, the hops in beer and the grapes or con-geners in wine.

## Monosodium Glutamate Headaches

A few years ago the 'Chinese restaurant syndrome' was de-scribed. It included headaches, often of the migraine type, sweat-ing, hairs 'standing up on the back of the neck', burning in the chest, face, jaw, body and trunk. Symptoms usually occur within fifteen to twenty minutes of eating. The trigger, monosodium glutamate, a flavour enhancer, is found in many products includ-ing dry-roasted peanuts, instant soups, instant gravies, some meat tenderizers and seasonings and some processed meats. Read labels carefully if you think you have had problems with this substance.

## Nitrate Headache

Nitrates produce dilation of blood vessels and in some people can produce a pounding headache. They have been used for cen-turies as a meat preservative. Some patients who take nitrate-containing drugs for angina complain of headaches.

Foods containing nitrates include:

tinned ham
hot dogs
corned beef
salami
bacon
pepperoni
smoked fish
sausages.

# SLEEP PATTERNS AND MIGRAINE

Lack of sleep can trigger migraine and oversleeping at weekends can also produce a migraine. This could be due to low blood sugar, the post-stress migraine response or caffeine withdrawal.[3]

## Post-stress Migraine

This is very common and usually happens at weekends. A fourteen-year-old boy who had a migraine attack every weekend starting on Friday evenings and lasting until midday Sunday became completely migraine-free when he was moved from a rigid grammar school to the local comprehensive school. Many businessmen have weekend migraines.

# CLUSTER HEADACHES

This is a rarer type of headache which is easily distinguishable from other types of headache. They are often called histamine headaches because it is histamine which causes the pain and inflammation associated with allergic headaches. Men are more prone to this than women and it is usually middle-aged men who are affected, although it can start as early as the mid-twenties. Alcohol drinkers and smokers are much more at risk or even non-smokers who have to sit in a smoke-filled room. The name comes from the fact that the headaches appear in 'clusters' and the victim is perfectly well between attacks, which last for six to eight weeks. Alcohol is well known to precipitate an attack in a known sufferer.

It is characterized by severe unilateral pain in the eye and temple, often occurring in the night, and can be so intense that the sufferer bangs his head on a wall. The face is flushed and hot and the eye on the affected side is swollen and bloodshot; the pupil is small and there is often profuse tearing. The affected nostril either streams with clear fluid or is swollen and blocked. Fortunately the pain is of quite short duration, easing within the hour and leaving a dull ache around the eye which can last for several hours. This can happen several times a day. Without treatment the pain can return daily for several weeks.

## Questions to Ask yourself

- Did your headaches begin after the age of twenty-five?
- Do your attacks occur at the rate of between one and six per day and continue for one to three months?
- Do you have eye and nose symptoms during the headache?
- Are you a smoker or drinker?
- Are you well between attacks?

## Treatment

Inhalation of oxygen can abort an attack of this type of headache and GPs are able to prescribe this on the NHS. A large cylinder is needed because the flow-rate must be seven litres per minute.[4]

Ergotamine tartrate can be used to prevent attacks although it is not without its risks and should not be prescribed for people with high blood pressure.

If you believe you have cluster headaches, it is essential to see your doctor to have the diagnosis confirmed; in addition, self-help methods to improve your general health can only be of value.

# MIGRAINE – THE HOLISTIC APPROACH

- Find the trigger.
- Boost your immune system and general health.
- Review your lifestyle and watch your stress levels.
- Look at your diet, alcohol intake, smoking habits, use of pre-scribed and over-the-counter drugs, and street drugs.
- Consider what you are opting out of when you have these migraines.
- Are you hanging on to negativity from the past?
- Are you full of pride and righteous indignation?
- Are your emotional needs being met?
- Are you afraid of death, of being alone?
- Do you ignore your spiritual needs?
- What about your feelings of self-worth?
- Investigate non-drug treatments.

Before you say 'but migraine is purely physical' – remember that **nothing is purely physical.**

# EMPULSE – NEW HOPE FOR SOME MIGRAINE SUFFERERS

Empulse has transformed the lives of many migraine sufferers. It is a simple, battery-operated device, a pulsed magnetic-field generator controlled by a microcomputer. It measures 4.5 × 4.5 × 1.5 cm and is worn twenty-four hours a day by the patient. It can be put under the pillow at night.

## How Does it Work?

The principle behind the treatment is that abnormal electrical impulses in the brain can cause physical symptoms and in some people correcting these abnormalities alleviates the symptoms. The conditions that the device has been found to be most successful with are migraine, ME, arthritis and back pain, insomnia, stress/tension, depression and allergies.

## The Development of Empulse

The theory of Empulse was developed by Stephen Walpole, an electronics engineer. As a result of a car accident in 1979 he began to suffer severe migraine and was told that there was no effective relief. In conjunction with a number of medical practitioners he began his research, which culminated in the development of what is now known as the Empulse device. There are now (1996) thirty-three practitioners, GPs and other health workers throughout the country using Empulse in their practices. They are all very enthusiastic about the treatment.

## What Does the Treatment Cost?

The device costs around £140, which is refundable if the patient does not benefit from it. Added to that is the consultation fee, which is usually between £20 and £40. Follow-up appointments are usually less and they may be weeks or months apart.

# What Happens during an Empulse Consultation?

The sufferer is required to attend a treatment centre where, after taking a detailed history, an analysis is made using a computerized brain frequency analyser. The analysis takes about five minutes (the full consultation takes a lot longer), and involves the patient wearing a comfortable headset linked to the analyser. A graph is produced showing the relative power of the signals received from the brain within the frequency bands considered to be important in respect of physiological conditions, as follows.

### Delta, 0.5–3.0 Hz★

Due to the fact that delta frequencies are associated with subconscious and unconscious states, deficiencies in this area would normally indicate a sleeping or short-term-memory and concentration problem.

### Theta, 3.0–7.0 Hz

Theta frequencies are mainly related to REM (Rapid Eye Movement) sleep. This is recognized as the area of brain activity that corresponds to creative, artistic and intellectual thought processes. It is also believed that biochemical processes are controlled by this frequency range. More than 70 per cent of migraine sufferers have deficiencies in the theta band.

### Alpha, 7.0–12.0 Hz

The primary function of alpha frequencies is in the control of muscular activity. The more alpha activity there is present, the more physically relaxed an individual is. Consequently, low levels in this frequency range often indicate stress, both physical and mental.

### Beta, 12.0–30.0 Hz

Beta is where nearly all thought processes occur, most sensory information is sent, changes in emotional states are seen and autonomic functions are controlled.

★Thank you to Russell Dick for this information.

## Migraine and Empulse

More than 70 per cent of migraine sufferers have deficiencies in the theta band, indicating that in many people a biochemical imbalance is the cause of the problem. In the remainder it can be a physiological problem, stress or perhaps a poor quality or low quantity of sleep. There are many types of migraine, and numerous different triggers associated with them, but it is the aim of the Empulse to treat the root cause rather than the symptoms. By doing this, the migraine attack is prevented from occurring. When the graph has been interpreted the Empulse is programmed to correct abnormal impulses. Follow-up visits consist of further reading and if necessary adjustments.

## Experiences of Some Empulse Users

The time I spent interviewing Empulse users was very uplifting. The relief in many of the patients' voices was overwhelming. One woman, who had been totally migraine-free for seven months and also relieved of chronic neck pain after a fourteen-year history of it, said she woke one morning in a state of dread with pain in her neck and a feeling of an impending migraine attack. She was in a panic until she realized her battery had run out! (There is a little light on the device which goes out when this has happened.) To her great relief, when the battery was replaced her symptoms vanished.

NOTE. Keep a spare battery!

### Woman of Fifty-three

History of migraine for twenty-six years; some relief given by Migril.

I am only affected by pain on the left side of my head. The

first sign of an attack is a tingling in the same small area at the top of my skull, roughly above my left eye. Within a short time the pain starts, and moves down the back of my head, through the bones behind my ear and down into my neck. At the same time the pain radiates forward down over my left forehead and around the left eye. The pain always takes the form of a thin line, as though made by a needle. If left unchecked (without Migril) the pain would steadily increase and last approximately four days, gradually tailing off but leaving me with a heavy pulse in my head at the original starting-point. This would last for a day. I have always had regular migraines, rarely missing even one week between attacks, but Empulse has changed this completely. I should also mention I was *always* aware of a feeling in that small area in my head, as though a migraine attack was always waiting to start.

## Man of Forty

History of migraine for eight years. Every migraine drug on the market was tried without effect. A little help was given by relaxation therapy.

I would wake up with that 'here-comes-a-migraine' feeling and within a few hours would have a thick head, and then pain down one side of my head going into my eye, nose, cheek, ear and neck. The arm on the same side would often go numb. The pain was severe enough to make me feel sick and I would usually vomit. Bright lights and noises were unbearable. This would go on for two to three days. During this time I could not work or eat, and slept only in snatches. When the pain eased I would feel weak and depressed for a couple of days.

Since using Empulse the attacks only last from a few

hours to a day, during which time if I move slowly I can cope with undemanding work or listen to music. I am much more confident now about my ability to cope with attacks and don't live in such dread of the next one.

## Woman of Thirty-seven

History of migraine for two years. Nurofen helps pain; homoeopathy helped a little.

The pain affects the left side of my face. It usually starts in my neck and comes up over my head, or starts with a funny feeling in the centre of my forehead or left eye. If I take Nurofen then the pain goes quickly. If the pain is left unchecked then I can be sick, and the pain becomes really severe. Then I can feel numb down the left side of my face and in my left arm. I have had one attack where there was no pain, just numbness down the left side.

Since using Empulse my sleeping pattern is better and I don't get so cross and shout so much. The migraine pain is less and has been shown to be associated with my menstrual cycle. I tend to have attacks around ovulation and menstruation.

## Man of Twenty-eight

History of migraine for five years. In the short term, helped by beta blockers, Deseril, Sanomigran.

The doctor said I have 'classical migraine'; I always know when an attack is imminent because I feel droopy for a couple of days. I drop things and my balance is affected. Then I get 'floaters', or things look oddly shaped or blurred. I feel very cold before the headache and hot when it is at full pitch. I often feel better after I have vomited or had diarrhoea. Strangely enough I often feel quite well after an attack with a 'cleansed' feeling.

After using Empulse I had to eat humble pie – I thought it was a lot of hocus pocus. Now the attacks are less severe and intervals between them are getting longer and longer. I feel more energetic and my wife says I am better tempered.

## Man of Thirty-seven

History of migraine for twenty years. Drugs: Sanomigran, propranolol, Imigran – Imigran works approximately two thirds of the time.

I experience a spreading pain over the head, concentrating after several hours on one side. Then the pain becomes acute behind the eye. Each attack lasts up to thirty-six hours unless Imigran works. If it does, the attack is over within two hours. The attack is often followed the next day by a second, often worse, attack on the other side – I call it the echo migraine. I usually get them about once a week but have tension headaches much of the time.

Unfortunately, Empulse did not work for me.

Practitioners have found that in some people where Empulse did not work initially, there was a good response after other conditions such as allergies or hormonal problems had been treated. For those who get immediate and continued freedom from migraine it seems like a miracle.

## SOURCES OF HELP

The British Migraine Association
178a High Road
Byfleet
Surrey KT14 7ED

The Migraine Trust
45 Great Ormond Street
London WC1N 3HD

To find your nearest Empulse practitioner contact:

Medical Devices and Instrumentation Ltd
17 Owen Road
Diss
Norfolk IP22 3ER
Tel. 01379 644234.

## REFERENCES

1. Walker, J., et al., 'Analgesic rebound headache: experience in a community hospital', *Southern Medical Journal* (Birmingham, Al.), 1993, Nov. 86 (11), 1202–5
2. Larson, Eric W., 'Migraine with typical aura associated with fluoxetine therapy', *Journal of Clinical Psychiatry*, 54, 6 (June 1993)
3. Couturier, E.G., 'The smart person will never sleep late: "weekend headache" due to late and insufficient intake of caffeine', *Ned Tijdschr Genceskd*, 137, 39 (25 September 1993)
4. Blau, J. N., *Understanding Headaches and Migraine*, Which? Books, 1991

## FURTHER READING

Sachs, Oliver, *Migraine*, Faber & Faber, 1970

## BIBLIOGRAPHY

Antony, M., 'Histamines and serotonin in cluster headaches', *Arch. Neurol.* 25 (11 Sept. 1971), 225–31
Ashton, C. H., 'Caffeine and health', *British Medical Journal*, vol. 295, no. 6609, p. 1293

Greden, John F., Victor, Bruce S., Fontaine, Patricia, and Lubetsky, Martin, 'Caffeine – withdrawal headache: a clinical profile', *Psychosomatics*, 21, 5 (May 1980)

Young, Sophie, 'Pilot study concerning the effects of extremely low frequency electromagnetic energy on migraine', *Journal of Alternative and Complementary Medicine*, October 1993 (Empulse)

# 7

# Headaches Caused by Sinus Problems

Television commercials would have us believe that all headaches with facial pain are due to sinus infections, and urge us to take their brand of antihistamine or decongestant. This is not so; there are numerous causes of facial pain with headaches. They include dental problems, temporo-mandibular joint (TMJ) problems and neuritis (nerve pains).

The sinuses are spaces in the bones of the skull which are filled with air from a small opening in the nose. The mucous membrane lining the nose is continuous with the lining of the sinuses and other structures connected with the nose, so infections in the nose can lead to infections of the eye, ear (and through the Eustachian tube), inner ear and the mastoid process of the temporal bone, throat, bronchi and, although very rarely, the meninges (the outer covering of the brain) by way of the olfactory nerve.

There are various causes of sinus problems; these may be categorized as allergic, acute infective or chronic.

## ALLERGIC SINUS HEADACHE

This is due to an allergic response inflaming the air inlet in the nose to the sinuses. It can be caused by inhalation of a substance (see pp. 104–5) which causes swelling in the delicate nasal mucosa, or by eating or drinking something which has the same effect. The resulting headache is known as a vacuum headache. It is unlike hay fever in that it only rarely involves streaming eyes and nose. It does not seem to be the effect of local irritation, with rapid onset of sneezing and so on. It is, however, possible that the action of chewing food may transmit allergens into the nasal cavity, thus provoking a response in the nose directly.[1]

## Characteristics

swelling inside the nose
difficulty with breathing through the nose
generalized headache, muzziness
dizziness
sudden mood change – anxiety, depression
pain over the cheek-bones and eyebrows, and at the base of the
    nose

The headache can be accompanied by:

rapid pulse
feeling weak and shaky
swelling around the eyes
hyperventilation
bloated abdomen and wind
fluid retention

It is possible that the lining of the gut swells in the same way as the lining of the nose. This could account for the feeling of 'everything stopping' in the abdomen. Constipation and bloating and difficulty in passing even a soft stool are common, although in some cases diarrhoea can be present. Often the first sign that symptoms are abating can be the passing of wind and movement in the gut.

Feelings of anxiety or panic, with pins and needles or heavy limbs are often reported when the nose is blocked. Rapid shallow mouth-breathing during the night brings on the symptoms of hyperventilation (see p. 163).

The symptoms may develop minutes after exposure or may take six or more hours to appear. Some symptoms such as restlessness and bloating may appear before the headache.

## Appearance
Pale, puffy-faced and tired.

# What to do to Relieve Symptoms

- If food intolerance has caused the reaction take a teaspoonful of bicarbonate of soda or, better still if you can get it, one teaspoonful each of bicarbonate of soda and potassium bicarbonate.* Drink plenty of water; as soon as you can, eat a bland meal, for example rice, pasta or something you know you can tolerate. For some reason this seems to 'turn off' reactions in some people.
- To reduce swelling in nose – steam inhalations, steamy bath or shower followed by cool shower. (Allergies are always worse when you are hot.)
- Some people find taking an antihistamine helps.
- Sodium cromoglycate nasal spray (available over the counter as Resiston) helps some people, although it seems more effective in preventing a reaction (see p. 106).
- Take a homoeopathic remedy or paracetamol for the headache.

*This is available from some chemists or you could try a health food store or nutritional supplier. 'Allergy Switch Off' is available from the Sanford Clinic – see Useful Adresses.

- Rest, with or without an ice pack (a packet of frozen peas wrapped in a thin cloth will do) on the head, forehead or over the bridge of the nose. Boots sell an ice pack with a cover.

## In the Longer Term

- Have food and chemical allergy testing. Your doctor might be able to help you. If not, see an alternative practitioner who is knowledgeable on this subject. If you cannot afford this, read about elimination/rotation diets and pay attention to your general health. Read a candida questionnaire. (See Shirley Trickett, *Coping with Candida*, Sheldon, 1994.)
- Watch out for stress – you are far more likely to have reactions when your body is already overtaxed.

## Case Histories

### Woman of Twenty-seven

I was unwell for several weekends while staying with a friend before I associated it with travelling by train. My income had gone up so I began to travel by train instead of the coach. At first I thought I was allergic to her cats but knew they had never bothered me before. The only difference I could pinpoint was travelling by train. I don't know whether it's the air-conditioning or something from the brake fluid (I loathe the smell), but it was definitely something on the train because I have not had it again since I went back to coach travel.

When I look back I remember feeling restless on the train and my nose felt uncomfortably dry. By the time I arrived at my friend's my eyes were puffy and I felt muzzyheaded and tired. A couple of times she asked me if I had been having late nights. During the evening my head would ache, I would feel bloated and as though I was retaining fluid before a period. I would also feel very thirsty. The next day my sinuses would feel sore and I often felt dizzy and weak. It cleared up after I had been home for a couple of days.

## Man of Forty-two

This man had a long history of what he called sinus problems. After years of ineffective treatment with antihistamines, decongestants and occasionally antibiotics he realized that his problem was not due to infections or an allergic reaction to an outside allergen but to some reaction in his body chemicals. The attacks were always after he had been overworking or after a stressful event. He asked his doctor if it were possible to get inflammation in his body as a result of stress. He got no reply to this and was given a prescription for a nasal spray. There was never any nasal discharge or post-nasal drip – just a blocked nose, which he felt was swollen inside.

It would start with a feeling of being uptight and vaguely depressed and I would have difficulty thinking. Then my nose would feel blocked, my head muzzy, with pains across my cheek-bones, and my stomach would feel bloated and uncomfortable. I would go off my food and feel unsteady on my legs. My neck and shoulders always felt very tense and my face would go pale and puffy. My wife said she always knew when it was coming on because I had dull red marks below my cheek-bones. I often felt as if I was going down with flu but there was never any sign of a temperature, although my face and head felt uncomfortably hot. The depression usually got worse and did not lift until the attack passed, which usually took three weeks no matter what I did. My sleeping was disturbed and I often woke up feeling slightly panicky, with pins and needles or a numb feeling in my arms.

The attacks became more frequent and my work and normally happy home life was being disrupted, so I had to slow down. I stopped working in the evenings, took a decent break at lunchtime and generally started to look after myself. Cutting down my workload caused me some anxiety at first and I had to be disciplined about delegating or leaving things to the following day. I also put the answering machine on in the evenings. Nagging from my wife helped. She was getting very fed up with me being below par. After about six weeks I felt the effect and realized I was achieving more although I was working fewer hours. I have only had one 'sinus' attack in the past year and that was after a hectic business trip to Canada.

# INFECTIVE SINUS PROBLEMS

Acute sinusitis is an infection of the lining of the nose and sinuses caused by bacteria, viruses or fungus (although this is not often looked for as a cause of sinus problems); it can spread to the throat and ears. It often appears about a week to ten days after a cold or flu as a secondary infection.

You can feel tired, lack concentration or have a feeling that your head is too heavy to be supported by your neck. Feeling vaguely anxious or depressed for no apparent reason, for a day or two before the attack really gets going, is common.

## Symptoms

fever

severe headache, facial pain, pain at the base of the nose, pain at the back of the neck and sometimes into the shoulders

dizziness

severe facial pain when you bend your head forward – this can also make you feel nauseated

blocked nose

dry throat, coated tongue

uneasy feeling in digestive tract

inability to think clearly

## Appearance

The face can look normal or swollen and can either be pale with red patches over the cheeks or be generally flushed. The nose can be swollen, with redness over the bridge. There is often considerable puffiness around the eyes (which can be bloodshot) and the neck can also look puffy. Some sufferers are sensitive to noise and light and most people with this infection feel generally very miserable.

## Treatment

The aims of treatment are:

to prevent the infection spreading to throat, ears and chest

to reduce the temperature and ease discomfort

to reduce the swelling in the nose so as to aid the discharge of mucus and allow air to flow into the sinuses.

If your symptoms do not respond to rest, aspirin or paracetamol, plenty of hot drinks and steam inhalations, see your doctor or homoeopath, particularly if your throat or ears are also involved. The doctor may prescribe an antibiotic.

## Avoiding the Unwanted Effects of Antibiotics

Antibiotics do not discriminate: when they kill bacteria they also kill off the useful bacteria which control the ecology of the gut and the result can be that fungi such as *Candida albicans* proliferate and cause symptoms such as bowel disturbances, a sore mouth, thrush and itching around the anus and genitals. These problems can be prevented or minimized by using antifungal preparations and avoiding foods such as sugar and yeast which encourage fungal growth (see Shirley Trickett, *Coping with Candida*, Sheldon, 1994).

## Steam Inhalations

These reduce swelling in the nasal passages and allow the drainage of mucus from the sinuses. Use one pint of near-boiling water with or without:

- one teaspoonful benzoin tincture (Friar's Balsam)
- a couple of menthol crystals
- five drops of Oil of Olbas (can be inhaled directly from the bottle or on a tissue).

Bend the head, covered with a towel, over the bowl and breathe in slowly through the nose until the steam has gone.

All the above are available from the pharmacist. Do not use them for babies or children.

## Essential Oils

Several oils, including pine, eucalyptus, lavender, ginger, peppermint and niaouli are helpful for sinusitis. NOTE. Essential oils are potent medicines and should be used with care during pregnancy and for children. Seek the help of an aromatherapist or follow the instructions in a book on aromatherapy.

## Ice Packs

An ice pack to the head or nape of the neck can be soothing. Use for twenty minutes in any one hour. (But see Note below.)

## Lavender Compress

Use five drops of lavender oil in bowl of warm water. Soak two thin cloths (small pieces of old cotton) in the bowl. Wring out one and allow to dry on the forehead; then replace with the second cloth.

NOTE. While the application of an ice pack can relieve some headaches, a cold substance in the mouth can actually cause a so-called 'ice-cream headache'. This headache is fortunately brief, though intense. When a cold substance touches the roof of the mouth many of the cranial nerves are affected and a dull throbbing pain can radiate all around the head. Children often cry out in pain at the first large spoonful of ice-cream. It can be avoided if the mouth is cooled slowly by eating small, well-spaced quantities. A biting wind can also produce a headache, usually in the forehead, temples or base of the skull.

## Acute Sinusitis – Quick Reference

- Seek professional help if the symptoms do not respond to rest, paracetamol and fluids.
- Keep in a warm atmosphere. Make the room steamy with wet towels on the radiator or an electric kettle. Germs in the nose breed more rapidly in cold conditions. The moist atmosphere will make it easier to breathe.
- If you have to go out in cold weather wear a hat and cover your nose and mouth with a scarf.
- Rest as much as possible.

- Use small tissues for blowing the nose and discard immediately. Wash hands.
- Take up to 3 g of vitamin C daily if your digestion can cope with it. If not, eat fresh fruit and vegetables.
- You will need your energy to fight the infection, so don't overload your digestion. Eat small, easily digested meals.
- Restock the gut with good bacteria.*

## Case Histories

### Man of Forty-three

Two weeks after an attack of flu I had acute sinusitis for the first time. It felt as bad as flu; I was utterly miserable. My face and head ached and I had a high temperature. I was given antibiotics and after about a week my nose streamed with a thick yellow discharge. This greatly relieved the pains in my head and face although I still felt weak and depressed. Part of the trouble was difficulty sleeping.

This is a typical experience of acute sinusitis as a secondary infection after flu or a cold.

### Woman of Thirty-three

Two years after I had stopped taking diazepam (Valium) I was very pleased with myself but was feeling run-down. (I had been on Valium for ten years and was originally prescribed it for exam nerves.) I was getting repeated sinus and ear infections which were really making me feel low and I

*Supplements containing acidophilus are available in health food stores but to be sure of a quality product it is better to order through a nutritional supplier. Biocare Ltd (see Useful Addresses) supply Replete, a special intensive seven-day programme to follow antibiotic usage.

was having a lot of sick leave. I had severe facial pain and could not look down at the keyboard, my concentration was nil and I felt dizzy and unreal. My ear discharged a lot and it dried around my ear and on my face like a salt deposit. It made the skin sore. It persisted in spite of several antibiotics. Eventually the doctor sent off a swab to the hospital. When the result came back he said he was surprised to find it was a fungal infection. I did not know at the time but learned later (from a health magazine) that long-term tranquillizer use can put a strain on the immune system and fungal infections after withdrawal are common. I was given anti-fungal drops and tablets and felt much better after a few days, although it did come back when the treatment stopped. I had to have two further courses of treatment.

## CHRONIC SINUSITIS

This is a debilitating condition which makes the sufferer feel miserable. The nose and sinuses are in a permanent state of inflammation and infection. This can give rise to the following symptoms:

headaches and facial pain
nose blocked or running with thick mucus
post-nasal drip – mucus discharging behind the nose
swollen nose and face
snuffling
loss of sense of smell
enlarged lymph glands in neck
recurrent ear, throat or chest infections
digestive problems caused by swallowing mucus
loss of appetite

general fatigue with aching muscles due to toxins
disturbed sleep
cough due to post–nasal drip.

## Treatment

The aims of treatment are:

to build up the immune system to enable it to cope with
infection
to reduce swelling in nose so as to allow mucus to drain
to prevent reinfection.

If this has been a long–term problem with you, ask your doctor for referral to an ear, nose and throat unit for investigations to rule out nasal polyps or any other condition. Nasal polyps are small grape–like swellings of the membrane formed by prolonged irritation.

- Avoid long–term use of nasal sprays, antibiotics, decongestants or antihistamines (see p. 105).
- Review your lifestyle – if you are stressed your immune system cannot recover.
- Review your diet – are you eating mucus–forming foods such as dairy produce and refined carbohydrate?
- Avoid smoky atmospheres.
- Have regular steam inhalations.
- Investigate the possible allergy/candida connection.
- Gargle with tea tree oil or Citricidal.★

★Tea tree oil supplier: Thursday Plantation, Illingworths, York House, York Street, Bradford BD8 0HR. Tel. 01274 488511.

Supplier of Citricidal: Penny Davenport, Nutrition Adviser, Woodlands, London Road, Battle, E. Sussex TN33 0LP. Tel. 01424 774103.

- Learn about nasal hygiene (pp. 91–2).
- Change your toothbrush frequently.
- Get as much fresh air as possible.
- Buy an ionizer (p. 186) for your bedroom.
- If you don't improve with self-help methods, seek help from complementary medicine.
- Try sleeping with more pillows.

## Case Histories

### Man of Thirty-five

After years of spraying my nose, and taking antibiotics and decongestants, I was fed up. The relief was always temporary and I was back to square one. I could cope when the mucus was draining but when I could feel my sinuses were full and nothing was happening I felt awful. All it took to bring on a headache was to look down at something on my desk. The pressure and pain in my face made me feel sick. It was after months of this that I booked ten sessions with a reflexologist. The advertisement said it was helpful for headaches and sinus problems.

By the seventh session nothing had happened and I felt really discouraged. I think the chap was feeling the same but he asked me to finish the course. I'm glad I did. In the middle of that week it was as though someone had turned a tap on. My nose poured with a thick bloodstained discharge. It went on for days. He asked me not to take anything and just to have steam inhalations. I felt wonderful. My head felt clear for the first time for years. That was two years ago. I have been back once for another course of treatment.

## Woman of Fifty-seven

I had recurrent ear infections after my fourth child was born and have had chronic sinus problems since. I have had X-rays and years of treatment from the doctor but it never seemed to clear completely. My sister suggested garlic capsules and cod liver oil. It worked wonders. I still have a bit of trouble in the winter but it is better than it has been for years. Some of my aches and pains have gone too.

## Man of Forty-five

Chronic catarrh had plagued me for years. Antibiotics and the nasal spray had stopped working. My digestion became a big problem and the hospital said it was irritable bowel syndrome. At the time I did not realize how this and the treatment I had been having for years for the sinus problem tied in together. The pills I was given for my gut did not seem to do anything and the high-fibre diet definitely made me worse. The whole of my abdomen was distended and I felt inflamed inside.

My wife had sent off to a candida helpline for information on thrush; she had had it off and on for years. There was a leaflet enclosed on irritable bowel syndrome. It was the first thing that had made sense. I changed my diet and sent away for the candida control packs.★ I felt a bit rough at first but it was worth it. Part of it, I think, was that it seemed to unblock my nose and swallowing the mucus down the back made me feel sick. When this drained I felt much better. I am on my third month of treatment and feel a different person.

★Suppliers of the candida control pack, Cantrol: Health Plus, P O Box 86, Seaford, E. Sussex BN25 4ZW. Tel. 01323 492 096.

This is a very common experience. Treating fungal overgrowth in the bowel often clears long-term ear, nose, throat and chest problems. It can also help chronic skin problems including psoriasis. While many doctors who practice nutritional medicine believe there is a direct link to fungal infections and psoriasis, conventional medicine favours the view that since the skin and gut come from the same part of the foetus, food intolerance is a more likely cause.[2] It is estimated that 25 per cent of eczema sufferers and 20–25 per cent of psoriasis sufferers are milk intolerant.[3] Many people on candida diets exclude all dairy products.

# GRAPEFRUIT-SEED EXTRACT – A NATURAL ANTIBIOTIC

Grapefruit-seed extract (Citricidal) is an inexpensive, safe addition to your medicine cabinet. It can be used for treating a host of common problems including sore throats, thrush, nappy rash, sinus infections, athlete's foot and much more. 'Studies from a list of prestigious institutes have demonstrated grapefruit-seed extract to be effective against over twenty disease-causing bacteria, more than thirty fungi, and a host of single-cell parasites' (Alan Sachs, *Beyond Nutrition*, Winter 1994). Dr Louis Parish, MD, an investigator for the US Department of Health and the FDA, who has treated many people with intestinal problems, including dysentery, believes that grapefruit-seed extract 'gives more symptomatic relief than any other treatment'.

It was discovered by a doctor and Einstein laureate physicist who specialized in finding natural remedies; fourteen years ago he discovered that when he threw grapefruit seeds on to his compost heap they did not rot. The extract he made from the seeds may turn out to be the most benign antimicrobial discovered so far.

One of the disadvantages of conventional antibiotics is that they also kill off helpful bacteria, such as bifidobacteria and lactobacilli, in the gut. After treatment with Citricidal the bifidobacteria was unaffected and the lactobacilli only slightly reduced. Even more remarkably, this natural product also kills some viruses. William Shannon of the Microvirology Division at the Southern Research Institute found it was effective against herpes simplex (cold sores) and one of the influenza viruses.

A South American laboratory, Interlab, has also found that Citricidal inactivated the measles virus, and the US Department of Agriculture found that it was effective against four animal viruses, including foot and mouth disease and African swine fever.

Other laboratory tests have shown that grapefruit-seed extract can kill many of the common pathogenic organisms including streptococci, staphylococci, salmonella, pseudomonas, giardia, lysteria, legionella, *Helicobacter pylori* and *Capylobacter jejuni*. Dr Leo Galland, who prescribes it for chronic candidiasis, has reported treatment failure in only two out of 297 cases, and considers it to be 'a major therapeutic breakthrough for patients with chronic parasitic and yeast infections . . .' (An information pack of laboratory test results, reports on the use of grapefruit-seed extract and a protocol sheet is available on request from Higher Nature Ltd, Burwash Common, East Sussex, TN19 7LX.)

## REFERENCES

1. Brostoff, Jonathan, and Gamlin, Linda, *The Complete Guide to Food Allergy and Intolerance*, Bloomsbury, 1989
2. *British Medical Journal*, 14 December 1968
3. ibid.

# 8

# Allergy-induced Headaches

## Allergic Reactions

These are a hypersensitivity to certain substances either inhaled, ingested, absorbed through the skin or manufactured in the body, for example, the toxins from invading bacteria or viruses. The immune system protects the body by trying to eliminate substances which it does not recognize (allergens), and an excessive reaction results in allergic symptoms such as swelling and overproduction of fluid. Common allergic reactions are seen in hay fever, asthma, eczema and nettle rash. These are well recognized, as are severe allergic reactions to one or two foods, and these have to be avoided throughout life, since they can produce severe breathing difficulties.

## What Happens during an Allergic Reaction?

A chemical called histamine released by the mast cells is overproduced and causes:

dilation of blood vessels
swelling in the linings of the airways – lungs and sinuses
increased fluid at the site of injury
increase in flow of tears and nasal secretions
increased production of stomach acid
itchy, inflamed skin.

# The Role of the Immune System

The healthier the immune system, the more able it is to cope with allergens. If the immune system is depleted through ill health, stress, poor diet, lack of exercise or overuse of drugs, including alcohol, the development of allergic reactions is much more likely. Often people say, 'Why is this happening? I seem to be allergic to so many things at the moment.'

## The Production of Antibodies

The production of antibodies by the immune system is vital to kill off invading micro-organisms or deal with certain substances. When an allergen is encountered for the first time, white blood cells known as lymphocytes are produced and attach themselves to other white blood cells known as mast cells. On the *second* encounter with the same substance the allergen binds to the antibodies on the mast cell, causing the release of chemicals called mediators which help to destroy the invader if it is a micro-organism. If it is a chemical the immune system cannot tolerate, an allergic reaction is the end result.

## The Importance of the Second Exposure

People with food intolerances need to understand that it is the second encounter with the allergen which causes the reaction. Hence, if you have become intolerant to wine and you have some at a dinner party you can feel fine but if you take it again the following day, even half a glass, you could have a reaction.

# Food and Chemical Intolerance

This condition does not produce the dramatic symptoms of severe allergy, and is sometimes called masked or hidden allergy. It is described in detail in Dr Richard Mackarness's book *Not All in the Mind* (Pan, 1977). Food intolerance is an inflammatory response by the body to foods which are eaten regularly. When they are stopped, cravings and other withdrawal symptoms can develop. This has been much more frequent in the past thirty years, and could be the result of the human immune system not being able to cope with junk foods, or to an increase in prescribed drugs and environmental pollutants. The diagnosis is not well recognized and is often confused with other conditions, particularly psychological problems. This is possibly because there are many symptoms which are not clearly defined. It is often treated as hypochondriasis.

# THE ALLERGY HEADACHE

Migraine can be triggered by certain foods and chemicals (p. 68); the offending substances seem to be the amine-rich foods such as cheese, chocolate or red wine (see p. 69), while those who suffer from food intolerances and hence headaches would be more likely to react to a much wider range of foods.

The typical allergy headache differs from migraine in that:

the pain is not localized – it is an 'all-over headache'
the pain is generally less severe
many of the accompanying symptoms do not appear in migraine attacks.

The sufferer often complains that the brain feels swollen, that they feel fuzzy or heavy-headed, they lose concentration and sometimes have feelings of unreality. Mood swings are also common and the sufferer can suddenly feel depressed and have a dull headache after eating an offending substance. Some people feel sleepy with this headache; others feel restless.

## Symptoms Which Can Accompany Allergy Headaches

flushing, sweating after meals
palpitations
itchy, sore eyes
bags or deep black shadows under eyes
earache, itching in ears
foul taste in mouth, loss of taste
sore mouth, mouth ulcers
swollen lips
recurrent sore throat
abnormal thirst
stuffy nose
sinus problems
tight chest
asthma
hives (nettle rash)
inflamed digestive tract
bloating
continuous dull abdominal ache
colicky pains
indigestion
constipation
diarrhoea
flattened stool
feeling of never having a complete bowel movement
itching anus
frequency of urine
urgency of stool
muscle or joint pain
heavy legs
feeling of the brain being swollen
irritability, outburst of rage

feeling of being 'spaced out'
anxiety or depression after eating certain foods
chronic fatigue
hyperactivity

### Predisposing Factors in Food and Chemical Intolerance

genetic influence
stressed immune system
environmental factors
harmful bacteria, candida overgrowth,★ parasites in the gut
drugs
inflammation in the gut★
damage to gut wall – 'leaky gut'★
lack of hydrochloric acid or enzymes
disturbance of pancreatic function
low levels of butyric acid made in the gut'

# ALLERGIC RHINITIS HEADACHES

## Hay Fever

Hay fever, caused by inhaling pollen, creates a vacuum headache: the blood vessels swell in the nasal passages and cut off the air supply to the sinuses. This tends to produce heavy or 'cotton-wool' headaches rather than severe localized pain. The eyes are itchy, red and swollen, and water profusely; the nose streams and is red and swollen. (The copious fluid is an attempt to wash away the offending pollen.) The throat is often red and scratchy. If the condition becomes chronic it can be complicated by infection.

★See Shirley Trickett, Coping with Candida, Sheldon, 1994, and The Irritable Bowel Syndrome and Diverticulosis, Thorsons, 1990.

With hay fever, unlike other forms of rhinitis not due to pollen, symptoms disappear in the autumn and winter months. Homoeopathy can be an extremely effective treatment for hay fever, as it deals with the constitution as well as the distressing symptoms. Taking the strain off the immune system by omitting additives from the diet has helped some people.[2]

## Other Inhaled Substances which may Cause Headaches

dust mites
animal hairs
brake fluid on trains
exhaust fumes
printers' ink
tobacco smoke
gas, oil, factory fumes
air fresheners
formaldehyde
fumes from chipboard furniture, synthetic carpets
   (the fumes from these decrease with time)
chemical inhalants from plastics, adhesives
flooring in shopping areas

## Chemical Allergy Headaches

These can be more severe than hay fever, probably because of toxins reaching the brain; profuse mucus production is not necessarily a feature.

Symptoms include:

dull, throbbing, generalized headache
restlessness

mood swings
inability to breathe through nose
vague nausea
swollen abdomen.

## What to Do

It is not always possible to exclude the substance affecting you from your environment. The first thing to do is to identify what substance is causing problems and if possible wear a protective mask, ventilate your working area and take frequent breaks in the fresh air. Work to build up your immune system (p. 100). As well as treating the symptoms, you must also build up your general health. See your doctor for referral to an allergy unit and possibly for a prescription for a non-sedative antihistamine, or look for a homoeopath.

# DRUGS FOR RHINITIS

Drugs only suppress the symptoms – they do not cure the condition. They can also give you more troubles than you started with, so caution is necessary. If you cannot eliminate the substance from your environment in the long-term it is better if you can be desensitized.

## Antihistamines

These are also known as H¹ blockers; they are the most widely used drugs in the treatment and prevention of allergies. They inhibit the activity of the mast cells and reduce the amount of histamine produced. Their most common use is in the treatment of hay fever or rhinitis from other causes, such as animal fur or dust, when it is impossible to avoid all contact with the allergen.

Older antihistamines such as Piriton (chlorpheniramine) have largely been replaced by newer ones, such as Seldane, Triludan and Boots antihistamine tablets (terfenedine), which are less sedating. It is important to note, however, that some users still report a sedative effect and care should be taken when driving, operating machinery or at other times when full concentration is needed. Other preparations available are Hismanal and Pollon-Eze (astemizole).

## Side-effects

Side-effects include dry mouth, blurred vision, weight gain and difficulty passing urine.

TAKE CARE! Antihistamines can increase the sedative effect of alcohol and of any drugs which have a depressant effect on the central nervous system, such as tranquillizers, sleeping pills and antidepressants. They can have the opposite effect in children and make them hyperactive.

# Sodium Cromoglycate

This is another mast-cell inhibitor which limits the production of histamine; it is also used to prevent asthma and allergic rhinitis. It should be started before the hay-fever season as it can take several weeks to be effective. Initially a local reaction (more sneezing) can occur but this passes off after a few days. This is the only reported side-effect except, very rarely, an asthma attack. The nasal spray Resiston is available over the counter. Sodium cromoglycate can also be given in capsule form for food allergies.

# Decongestants

These reduce swelling in the nose in rhinitis and dilate the air passages in asthma. When the delicate mucous membranes are irritated, the blood vessels enlarge and increased amounts of fluid are produced. The result is the production of more mucus, which can be a breeding ground for micro-organisms. Decongestants allow the mucus to drain more freely. There are risks associated with these drugs, so if your symptoms are not too severe try steam inhalations with or without menthol crystals, Oil of Olbas (available from any chemist), eucalyptus or tincture of benzoin (Friar's Balsam).

## Common Decongestant Drugs

*phenylpropanolamine*, available as Mucron, Sinutab and Triogesic (with paracetamol); these can have a mild diuretic effect and can reduce appetite

*pseudoephidrine hydrochloride*, available as Sudafed

*ephedrine nasal drops* – these are the safest nasal drops in this group (sympathomimetic drugs)[3]

*xylometazoline nasal drops*, available as Otrivine.

NOTE. These nasal sprays should be used for a maximum of seven days to avoid any risk of rebound nasal congestion.

## Side-effects

Drugs which contain ephedrine and pseudoephedrine taken orally stimulate the sympathetic nervous system (p. 27) and for this reason are more likely to cause increased heart-rate and trembling. People with heart and blood-pressure problems, over-active thyroid glands or anxiety states should avoid these drugs. They are also unsuitable for people on monoamine-oxidase inhibitors (MAOI antidepressants).

## Rebound Congestion

When decongestants are stopped after being abused or used for long periods there can be an overreaction in the tissues due to the dilation of the blood vessels. Very careful use and gradual withdrawal is essential with these drugs in order to avoid chronic damage to the nasal mucosa.

## How Decongestants Are Used

This can be by nasal drops or sprays (local or topical action), or by mouth as tablets. Topical use is safer since the drug is poorly absorbed.

**Caution: if you are on any medication check with your doctor or pharmacist before you buy any antihistamines, nasal decongestants or cold cure preparations.**

# Case History

## Man of Thirty

I started getting hay fever when I was about ten years old. Life was a misery every summer. Five years ago I had my first attack of acute sinusitis. Life seemed just one round of either hay fever or sinus problems. I was worried about taking so many antibiotics and in spite of decongestants I felt blocked up most of the time and the headaches were getting me down. My girlfriend persuaded me to see her homoeopath. I have to admit I was sceptical at first. It was right in the middle of the hay-fever season. Within a week I had improved enough to make me want to continue with the treatment. I went for three months. I noticed a big difference when the cold weather came. It was the first winter for five years that I had not had repeated sinus infections. The following summer I had a mild bout of hay fever at the beginning of the season and went back for more treatment. I realize now I should have had treatment before the pollens started flying. I had very little trouble for the rest of that summer and have not had any problems since. The homoeopath also gave me a diet – no dairy produce and lots of vegetables and fruit. I think this helped too. I eat cheese from time to time now but I have kept off milk.

# OTHER APPROACHES TO TREATING RHINITIS

## Allergy Testing

Your doctor can refer you to the allergy department of an NHS hospital if you have respiratory symptoms (asthma, hay fever); the allergen causing you trouble can then be identified and treated by desensitization. Some hospitals also investigate and treat food intolerances.

If you find your doctor unwilling to accept your suspicions that food or chemical intolerance could be your problem, you may want to seek out a private clinic with a doctor who specializes in nutritional medicine. Other options are to find an alternative practitioner who is knowledgeable on the subject. (Many are.) If you have to rely on self-help, follow an elimination diet to find out what is affecting you. A colon cleansing programme★ plus nutritional supplements can help to build your immune system. Chapter 13 deals with other ways of boosting the immune system.

## The Skin Prick

In order to test for allergies, drops of liquid containing the common allergens are placed on the skin, which is then pricked

★See Shirley Trickett, *Irritable Bowel Syndrome and Diverticulosis*, Thorsons, 1990.

or scratched. If the patient is sensitive to the substance, inflammation of the area — known as the weal-and-flare response — develops. This is a standard test for inhaled allergens such as pollens and dust, but is unreliable for food intolerances. Sublingual drops (drops placed under the tongue) are also used to identify allergens and they are used in dilute concentrations for desensitization treatment.

## Intradermal Injections

These are more reliable; they go deeper into the skin than the prick. If the person is not allergic to the substance a small weal which soon disappears is produced. In a positive reaction the weal increases in size and becomes white and hard.

## Neutralization

This treatment is based on finding a dilution of the offending substance which will 'turn off' the allergic reaction by its influence on the immune system. A simple explanation of this can be found in Dr Richard Mackarness's book, *A Little of What You Fancy* (Fontana, 1985).

It is not known why neutralization therapy works, but it seems to have close parallels with the homoeopathic principle of like curing like — that is, the correct dilution of whatever the body considers a poison effecting a cure.

## Enzyme-potentiated Desensitization

A mixture of food extracts plus an enzyme is applied in a plastic cup to a scratch on the skin. Desensitization is presumably effected in the same way as in neutralization. This method of treatment is only needed about once every three months, and then less and less often as the immune system recovers. You are more likely to find this method in a private nutritional-medicine clinic.

## Kinesiology

Kinesiology or muscle testing is a simple and popular technique used by some doctors and many alternative therapists. It is based on muscle-testing techniques through which weaknesses are identified and treated. An antigen is placed on the surface of a patient's body (usually the abdomen), and certain muscles are tested for strengths and weaknesses. This is painless and effective, and the results are known immediately. Once the allergens are identified, homoeopathically prepared drops are administered, made from the offending substance, and this is usually given over a week, or two weeks if the allergy is persistent. These drops de-sensitize the patient and he/she is usually able to resume being in contact with the offender without any further problems. Usually one or two major allergens are found and once these are treated, the minor allergies usually clear up of their own accord. A full case history is taken before the testing begins.

### Case History

Jane, a twenty-nine-year-old divorced woman with two children, complained of migraines which started when she was twenty-three. She was getting them approximately twice per week and her work was being seriously affected. She brought with her small samples of food that she ate daily or nearly every day. She had stopped chocolate, cheese and red wine about three years previously but she still developed the migraines. I began to test her muscles for strengths and weaknesses. When I tested her with sugar and coffee, I noticed an immediate weakness in her muscle. She was amazed. She then had to avoid all sugars and coffee for a week while she took the desensitizing drops. After three weeks I re-tested her and found the weakness had disappeared. So, very slowly, she reintroduced sugars and coffee into her diet and there has been no recurrence of her migraines.

For further information on kinesiology contact Mr Donald Harrison, Ffynnonwen Natural Therapy Centre, Llangwyryfon, Aberystwyth, Wales SY23 4EY.

★

Thank you to Hazel White-Cooper and R. S. Hom, 18 Wilmington Close, Tudor Grange, Kenton Bank Foot, Newcastle upon Tyne, NE3 2SF, for the information on kinesiology.

# FOOD ALLERGY

## Food Intolerance: the Major Offenders

A study reported in the *Lancet*[4] showed that the main food allergens in adults were wheat, corn, dairy products, coffee, tea and citrus fruits. Infants are more likely to react to milk, soy and beef.[5] Symptoms in older children are often due to milk products, too much sugar, junk foods, food colourings and additives.

## Food Rotation

The principle of this is a diet involving rotation and diversification of food. You are most likely to become intolerant of foods you have eaten all your life. Food rotation allows the immune system to recover, by not bombarding it with the same allergen every day. Some people react to so many foods that they could not possibly exclude them all because they would become malnourished, so they eat most things but only once in four days.

The body seems to be able to cope with this and many people do well on it. It is tedious: it involves eating everything to do with the cow (dairy produce and beef) on one day and everything connected with sheep (lamb, lamb's liver, ewe's milk yogurt) on another day, and so on, and also a different grain, vegetable and fruit on every fourth day. This is a much sounder nutritional approach than eliminating several foods from your diet permanently, because, if you eat them daily, you can develop intolerances to new foods in the diet which do not initially cause a reaction. However, caution is needed, for long periods on very restricted diets can lead to vitamin and mineral deficiencies.

# THE EFFECTS OF FOOD AND CHEMICAL INTOLERANCE ON CHILDREN

failure to thrive
vomiting
diarrhoea
constipation
headaches
hyperactivity
aggression
mental dullness
recurrent ear, nose and throat problems
black circles under eyes
itchy nose
sleep disturbances
bed-wetting
excessive thirst

In an observational study,[6] all cases of a group of children suffering from symptoms of food allergies showed evidence of deficiencies of lactobacillus and bifidobacterias combined with enterobacteriaeae (harmful bacteria) overgrowth.

## FOR MORE INFORMATION

Action Against Allergy
43 The Downs
London SW20 8HG

Hyperactive Children's Support Group
59 Meadowside
Angmering
Littlehampton
West Sussex BN16 4BW

## REFERENCES

1. Neesby, Torben, 'Butyric acid complexes – a new approach to food intolerances', *Biomed Newsletter*, 1, 2 (Feb. 1990)
2. Freedman, B. J., 'A diet free from additives in the management of allergic disease', *Clin. Allergy*, 7 (1977), 417–21
3. British National Formulary, 27 (March 1994)
4. Alun-Jones, V. A., et al., 'Food intolerance: a major factor in the pathogenesis of irritable bowel syndrome', *Lancet*, 2 (1982), 1115–17
5. Jenkins, H. R., et al., 'Food allergy: the major cause of infantile colitis', *Annals of Allergy*, 153 (October 1984)
6. Kuvaeva, I., et al., 'Microecology of the gastrointestinal tract and the immunological status under food allergy', *Nahrung*, 28, 6–7 (1984), 689–93

## FURTHER READING

Magrath, Amy, *One Man's Poison – The 'Glucose' Factor*, available from Cirrus Associates, SW (see Useful Addresses). A mother's struggle to identify the glucose factor in carbohydrate, turning her children from unhealthy 'devils' into healthy 'angels'

Katahan, M., *The Food Rotation Diet*, Bantam, 1986

Brostoff, Jonathan, and Gamlin, Linda, *Food Allergy and Intolerance*, Bloomsbury, 1989

Rothera, Ellen, *Perhaps It's an Allergy*, Food & Chemical Allergy Association, 1988

Mumby, Keith, *The Food Allergy Plan*, Unwin, 1985

Paterson, Barbara, *The Allergy Connection*, Thorsons, 1985

# 9

# *Headaches Caused by Jaw Problems*

The temporo-mandibular or jaw joint is situated just in front of the opening in the ear. You can feel the movement if you press your finger firmly in front of your ear and move your jaw up and down. The muscles of this joint can be damaged by tension in the jaw, the joint being out of alignment, teeth-grinding or arthritis in the joint. The pain arises from stress in the muscles or joint, or from inflammation.

This problem is much commoner than you might think: an estimated seventy-five million people in the United States have TMJ problems,[1] nine out of ten people with tension headaches also suffer from TMJ problems.[2] TMJ problems are often overlooked or misdiagnosed.

## The Importance of the Jaw Joint

The jaw acts as a centre of body balance. When the jaw is in the correct position it allows the head to rest comfortably on the neck. If the lower jaw is forced out of place the head will be thrown out of balance and all the muscles supporting it will have to strain in order to keep it in position on the neck. We have seen earlier that tension in the neck muscles can send a message of tension to the whole body. It is not surprising, therefore, that the symptoms of a misaligned jaw go far beyond local pain.

# THE TMJ SYNDROME

The syndrome may involve the following symptoms:

    headaches which are usually unilateral and can be severe
    waking up with a headache
    pain in the joint itself, lower jaw, upper jaw, forehead, face,
        throat muscles, behind the eyes, in the temple, scalp, tongue,
        shoulders and neck
    stiffness or numbness in face or scalp
    sore eyes, sometimes with swelling
    one eye higher than the other
    mouth on affected side turned up
    abnormal wear in teeth on one side
    nocturnal teeth-grinding (bruxism)
    laborious chewing over meals or bolting meals without chew-
        ing, with resulting digestive problems
    leg shorter on affected side
    swelling in face
    grating or clicking in joint when chewing
    pain in ear when chewing
    feeling of pressure in ear or hissing, roaring or ringing noises
    sensitivity to noise; easily startled by noise
    restricted movement: difficulty opening mouth wide or mov-
        ing jaw from left to right or back and forth
    tingling in fingertips
    recurrent sinus, ear, nose and throat infections.

# How Does the Jaw Become Malpositioned?

## Genetic Influence

We are often built asymmetrically. For example, one leg can be shorter than the other and teeth may erupt irregularly. Since the teeth determine the position of the jaw, uneven teeth will not offer the full support that the jaw needs.

## Nutrition and Chewing Habits

These are important not only for the developing teeth but also to maintain the necessary bite. Children who suck their thumbs or hang on to their dummies or bottles too long may push their teeth out of position. Others clench or grind their teeth during stress. Adults do this too.

## Other Causes

Injury to the head and jaw, and holding the jaw in tense attitudes such as 'setting the jaw' in anger or holding it tense when on the telephone. Most TMJ problems are muscle-contraction or tension induced.

# Stress and the Jaw

The jaw is often the focus for stress-related habits such as:

   jaw-jutting
   pencil-chewing, nail-biting, continual gum-chewing
   nocturnal teeth-grinding
   propping jaw on cupped hands
   poor posture.

These actions cause the muscles to go into spasm and circulation is impeded. This causes malnourished areas of tissue which become painful trigger spots.

## Things to Consider

- Did your headaches begin after dental treatment?
- Do your dentures fit well?
- Did you have your teeth straightened as a child?
- Are your headaches immune to drugs?
- Does prolonged chewing bring on a headache?
- Is there tenderness in the muscles around the jaw?
- Does your jaw veer to one side when you let it hang?
- Can you insert the first three knuckles of your fingers into your mouth when it is as wide open as possible?
- Have you got missing teeth?
- Is one eyebrow higher than the other?
- When you gently clench your teeth, does the pressure feel the same at both sides?
- If you make an imprint by biting into a thick slice of soft bread are the indentations shallower on one side than the other?

## Become Aware of Your Jaw

There is no need for the teeth to come together except when chewing or swallowing. Train yourself to place the tip of the tongue behind the front teeth. It is impossible to jaw-clench when the tongue is in this position. Be aware of how you are chewing – use both sides of your jaw. Notice what happens to your jaw when you are talking. Are you thrusting it out – does it tense up?

## Treatment

### Professional Help

Pain from TMJ problems can only be relieved by the jaw being repositioned correctly, either by dental work or by an occlusal splint made by an orthodontist. This will correct your bite and allow the tense muscles to relax. This should have a dramatic effect on your headaches. Any other measure taken will be of limited value until the mechanics are corrected. Once the normal circulation to the head has been established you should have fewer sinus, ear, nose or throat infections.

### What Else Can I Do?

- Relax more!
- Treat the pain with analgesics.
- If you can, seek help from a cranial osteopath, osteopath, masseur, acupuncturist, shiatsu practitioner or any other pain-relief technique.
- Massage the tight muscles regularly yourself.
- Learn which essential oils help pain.
- Learn which acupressure points help the pain.
- See which helps pain most – the application of warmth or cold. Boots and the Body Shop have jelly packs which can be either heated or chilled.
- Do regular neck-stretching exercises.
- Support your chin when you yawn.
- Be aware of how you are holding your head.
- If you can afford it, have Alexander lessons (p. 231).

### TMJ Syndrome and Stress

The TMJ syndrome is generally associated with spasm in the muscles of mastication as a result of physical and/or psychological stressors.[3] It would make sense, therefore, to include relaxation therapy in your treatment even if you have been given an occlusal splint (see above). Many people who have had stress management as their only treatment have done well.

## Case Histories

### Woman of Forty-two

Two of my lower molars had to be capped. Both had temporary fillings; unfortunately because I had to go away and then because I was ill I had to miss several appointments. For a period of about six months I had no bite on that side; the teeth were reduced to a fraction of their normal size. It was not until I had been having headaches, numbness and stiffness in the jaw, and pain in my scalp and face for some time, that I realized the problems were caused by the jaw. My neck and shoulders felt permanently in spasm. I also had three attacks of sinusitis in that six months. My dentist confirmed my jaw was out of true and said that if the symptoms did not disappear when the crowns were completed he would make me a soft splint to wear at night and when I was working. He showed me some stretching exercises to do and told me to apply warmth to the jaw and neck. I asked my husband to massage my neck and shoulders before I went to bed. That seemed to help but the headaches did not go until a few weeks after the crowns were in place.

### Man of Thirty-seven

It was my osteopath who referred me to the dental unit. I am very glad he did. I was given a splint to wear at night and if I felt tense. It worked like magic: the headaches vanished.

I wish I had known about these splints years ago. It has made such a difference to my life. I don't wear it all the time now; only when I am under pressure.

## Woman of Twenty-nine

I had spent years changing my diet, doing yoga and hunting for something that would help my migraine attacks, but nothing seemed to work. I saw a piece in a migraine newsletter on TMJ as a precipitating factor in migraine. It made sense to me. My brother (another migraine sufferer) and I had both had our teeth in braces for years when we were kids. I went rushing off hopefully to the doctor to be referred to a consultant but he said he thought it an unlikely cause of migraine and just gave me some painkillers. My dentist was more helpful. He pressed inside my mouth and around my jaw and neck and said he thought there was inflammation in the muscles and it would do no harm to have it checked, although he also said it might not be the cause of the migraine. He referred me to an orthodontist who said I did have a problem jaw and he could not understand why I had left it so long. He made me an occlusion splint and it has helped enormously. I still get the odd migraine attack but they are a shadow of what they were.

# Just How Effective are Occlusal Splints? (*from* Factsheet no. 4, *Migraine Trust*)

Since the early 1980s there have been fairly frequent claims of the efficacy of certain dental treatments, usually in relation to alterations of the 'bite' for the treatment of migraine. Claims of success, including one bold statement that 90 per cent of migraineurs need not suffer, have been met with scepticism in many quarters, not least the dental profession itself. There was a dearth of results from properly controlled research and most of the claims were based on hearsay, or 'clinical experience'. However, in the late 1980s a few results appeared in refereed journals. The oral medicine department of Glasgow Dental School in which I worked has a large group of patients, some of whom seemed to have experienced marked improvement following the provision of a small plastic appliance or splint. The device covered either the upper or lower teeth, was only worn at night and appeared to work best in those whose attacks of headache started on waking from sleep or soon afterwards. The appliance or 'splint' separates the teeth, and in theory allows the jaws to find the most comfortable position. It may also prevent habits such as tooth-grinding or clenching which can act as headache triggers (although not necessarily for migraine).

This experience suggested that there was some benefit to migraineurs which, if it was targeted correctly, could improve the quality of life of quite a lot of people. However, the complexity of individual migraine histories meant that it was difficult to be sure whether the reduction was in actual migraine attacks, or other headache types, for example tension headaches which were occurring in combination. The problem of a 'placebo-effect' of splint wearing must also be addressed.

With the help of a grant from the Migraine Trust, I was able to set up a clinical trial to investigate the potential benefits of splint wearing. About forty people who had been diagnosed as migraineurs by their general practitioners or neurologists were selected to take part. To take part in the trial all the participants had to experience attacks frequently (at least twice a month) and to report at least half of their attacks to begin on waking or soon afterwards. As the splint was only for night wear, it was important to target those whose attacks were triggered during the night, and this was the group who had previously been reported as most likely to benefit. At this stage the accuracy of the original diagnosis was not particularly important as each attack was to be diagnosed objectively during the trial.

All of the participants recorded the details of each attack on a separate form for a ten-week spell before treatment, and were then given an active splint or a placebo splint (which did not cover the teeth) on a random basis for another ten-week period. Those who wore the placebo were given an active splint to wear for a further period of ten weeks. During all of this time the patients recorded the details of every attack, which made a diagnosis possible for each one. All the forms were then analysed blind and a diagnosis of each attack was made, by rigidly applying the most recent diagnostic criteria, and its duration calculated.

The results produced some interesting findings. Firstly, many of those who suffered from migraine attacks also suffered from tension headaches. About a quarter of the patients who completed the trial showed a measurable benefit; in some cases it was very marked, but the biggest reduction tended to occur in those who suffered frequent tension-type headaches. Where both tension-type headaches and migraines occurred together it was the tension attacks which usually showed most reduction. Statistical analysis suggested that attacks of migraine with aura (classical migraine) were unaffected. Migraine without aura (common migraine) appeared to be reduced but the reduction was only slightly greater than would be expected by chance, and even using the available diagnostic criteria separating these from tension headaches is not always easy. Tension headaches on the other hand showed a marked reduction, in some quite dramatic. Two patients who had suffered almost daily headaches saw them almost completely eliminated.

Unfortunately the original promises of a wonder cure for migraine do not seem to hold. The successes in treating migraine in the past may have been due to the elimination of more frequent tension headaches which were occurring alongside attacks of migraine. However, we should not underestimate the benefits of this treatment. Many migraineurs' lives are made even more miserable by frequent, wearing, tension headaches, which occur in addition to their attacks of migraine.

For a proportion of these people, particularly those who often wake up with headaches, an occlusal splint may provide some relief.

J. G. STEELE
Department of Operative Dentistry
Newcastle Dental School

## REFERENCES

1. Gelb, Harold, *Killing Pain without Prescription*, Thorsons, 1983
2. Dick, Russell, 'The Temporomandibular Joint', available from The Croft, Durham Rd, Birtley, Chester-le-Street, Durham DH3 1LY
3. Henderikus, J. Stam, McGrath, Patricia A., and Brooke, Ralph I., 'The treatment of temporomandibular joint syndrome through control of anxiety', *Journal of Behavioural Therapeutics and Experimental Psychiatry*, 15, 1 (1984), 41–5

## BIBLIOGRAPHY

Morse, D. R., 'Stress and bruxism', *J. Human Stress*, 8, 43–54

# Low Blood Sugar and Headaches

## What is Hypoglycaemia or Low Blood Sugar?

The food we eat is processed and enters the circulation as a form of sugar. By this route all cells receive the fuel necessary for normal functioning. The pancreas (p. 33) secretes the insulin necessary to metabolize carbohydrate, and unless there is diabetes or, less commonly, an inherited tendency to have faulty carbohydrate metabolism, this system works well. Careless eating habits, high levels of anxiety and taking or withdrawing from certain medications can also give rise to hypoglycaemic symptoms. There are three types of hypoglycaemia: reactive, diabetic and organic.

### Reactive Hypoglycaemia

Reactive hypoglycaemia is by far the most common type. It is what it suggests: the body is reacting to the way it is being treated. The pancreas is being overtaxed by a high sugar/refined carbohydrate diet, missed or late meals, alcohol, caffeine, nicotine and other drugs (mentioned later), or stress. This type of hypoglycaemia responds to self-help methods such as diet and stress reduction.

Some foods, irrespective of their carbohydrate content, can produce an abnormally high or low blood sugar if the person is intolerant to them.[1] If your symptoms do not respond to the hypoglycaemic eating plan (see below), then you would do well to investigate food intolerances. You could start by cutting out the main allergens: wheat, dairy products and citrus fruit.

## Diabetic Hypoglycaemia

When a diabetic takes too much insulin the result is a dramatic drop in the blood sugar level.

## Organic Hypoglycaemia

This can be the result of an over- /under-active thyroid and would need to be investigated by your doctor. It can also occur after a partial gastrectomy. A rarer cause is organic disease of the pancreas or liver.

# Diabetes

This condition develops when the pancreas fails to secrete enough insulin to cope with the carbohydrate it is presented with. The result is that the sugar cannot be broken down and used by the body. The blood sugar levels become too high, *hyper*glycaemia, and sugar is excreted in the urine. Without treatment the sufferer would quickly become dramatically ill. Treatment consists of insulin injections/drugs and a diet with a measured daily amount of carbohydrate to meet the energy needs of the person. If the diabetic is given too much insulin or if he fails to eat the required amount, his blood sugar level drops and he becomes *hypo*glycaemic.

Many doctors believe that low blood sugar symptoms are of importance only in diabetics. Others, particularly those who work in nutritional medicine, believe that hypoglycaemia is a much neglected condition responsible for many of the chronic health problems which plague modern man. The digestive system in man is built for the slow absorption of complex carbohydrates, such as whole grains, vegetables, fruit, protein and fat. This gives the body a steady supply of glucose during the day and enough to last through the night during rest. The quick sugar fixes of the modern diet cannot do this. The constantly overworked pancreas produces an excess of insulin and the body reacts with a multitude of symptoms.

# WHEN THE BLOOD SUGAR LEVELS ARE LOW

*Symptoms*

- fatigue
- irritability
- headaches
- migraine
- dizziness
- fainting
- blurred vision
- twitching of muscles around the eye
- poor concentration
- forgetfulness
- anxiety
- panic attacks
- phobias
- depression
- wakefulness
- waking between 2.30–4.30 a.m.
- feeling of inner shaking
- cold hands and feet
- numbness
- joint and muscle stiffness

little desire for breakfast

food cravings, particularly sweet foods or drinks

alcohol craving

excessive smoking

allergies

epilepsy in susceptible individuals

This is an awesome list of symptoms. It could be questioned whether it is possible for such a multitude of ills to stem merely from hypoglycaemia caused by careless eating habits or by an exhausted nervous system. However, the disappearance of these symptoms, many of which might have been very long term and resistant to all other treatments, in people who have adhered to the diet given below, cannot be questioned. (For full explanations of why these symptoms develop, see Martin Budd, *Low Blood Sugar (Hypoglycaemia): The Twentieth Century Epidemic?*, Thorsons, 1981.)

The above symptoms appear in other conditions, particularly nervous problems. Anxiety may be characterized by:

sweating

palpitations

trembling

headaches

digestive upsets

changes in appetite

blood sugar problems

urinary problems

skin problems

neck and shoulder tension

dizziness

ringing in the ears

blurred vision

sinus problems

backache
wobbly legs
tight chest
overbreathing
difficulty swallowing
loss of interest in sex
insomnia
waking around 5 a.m.
irritability
confusion
restlessness
hopelessness
hyperactivity
lack of concentration
rapid speech
rapid thoughts
paranoia
phobias
feelings of gloom and doom
morbid thoughts
crying easily
laughing inappropriately
fainting
attention seeking
suicidal thoughts.

It is not surprising that there are many common symptoms in these two lists, and it is also understandable that both lists are so long. If the nervous system is under strain every system in the body is affected, whether the cause is worry or low blood sugar problems. People often ask why they get dramatic psychological symptoms (mood swings, panic, depression) if they skip meals, when they can still function physically: 'I'm not normally a nervous person.' The answer is that the muscles can utilize fat and protein to keep going in the absence of sugar, but the brain cannot. It relies entirely on a form of sugar to function, so confusion, headaches and so on are often the first symptoms of hypoglycaemia to appear.

It would be unwise, however, to assume your problems are necessarily due to hypoglycaemia. No matter how closely you identify with the list of symptoms, since many of the same symptoms appear in other conditions a medical check-up is necessary. If, on the other hand, you have seen a doctor and he maintains that it's just your nerves, you could still be greatly helped by following the diet principles described below.

## Is It an Illness?

Hypoglycaemia is not an illness but merely a reversible state. The treatment consists simply in changing the diet – if the symptoms, headaches, panic attacks, and so on disappear with careful eating, they are due to hypoglycaemia; if they don't, they are not. The following is taken from my book *Coping with Panic Attacks*:

I have seen hypoglycaemia in a clinical setting on a diabetic ward and also in the community when working with people with anxiety and addiction problems. In the latter groups, perhaps the condition could more accurately be called unstable blood sugar levels rather than low blood sugar levels because symptoms can occur when the blood sugar levels are within normal limits. It would appear that it is sudden drops which cause the problems rather than the blood sugar level being abnormally low. It is interesting to note that blood taken whilst patients were actually having panic attacks was on the lower end of the scale but never actually below normal, and yet their symptoms responded very dramatically to a diet designed to keep the blood sugar levels stable.

After seeing hundreds of people improve, here and in America, when following a low blood sugar eating plan (which needs to be a lot more than just sensible eating), I feel it has a huge part to play in the management not only of anxiety, but also of migraine, PMT and some types of asthma.

Whilst I see it as an important part of treatment, I also feel strongly that the approach to it should be one of common sense. In the absence of organic disease, glucose-tolerance tests are not only a waste of time, but can also make the patient feel very unwell for several days.

I see the answer as very simple: if the symptoms are coming from unstable blood sugar levels, they will begin to respond to diet within a few days. If the patient has not seen a dramatic improvement within three months, then it is not a blood sugar problem.

In my work in the community over the past twelve years, it has been a great joy to see so many 'no breakfast, sandwich lunch, large evening meal' eaters reduce their adrenalin levels, lose so many of their headaches and anxiety symptoms, and become confident and in charge by simply stopping their blood sugar levels from kangarooing.

## Low Blood Sugar – Shall I Go to the Doctor?

Unless you feel you have developed low blood sugar symptoms since you have been on a prescribed drug it is probably a waste of time to go to your doctor. My experience of the general medical reaction to this problem is: 'Yes, it is hypoglycaemia – drink sweet tea!' or 'No, only diabetics get that when they have too much insulin; you are just anxious.'

I quote now from my letter to the *Relaxation for Living Newsletter*. This was written in response to the profession being worried about lay people using the term hypoglycaemia. There was also some denial that the control of low blood sugar levels was an appropriate part of anxiety management. I was puzzled by this because I feel that it is necessary to explore all avenues by which the overproduction of adrenalin could be controlled.

We have seen that when the body is under stress the circulation is affected and the result is palpitations, missed heartbeats and so on. In addition to the expected anxiety symptoms there are some which are more specific to changing blood sugar levels. These are dull headaches, inner trembling but no visible shaking, sugar craving, waking between 2 a.m. and 4 a.m. alert, anxious and sometimes very hungry, low energy mid-morning and mid-afternoon, twitching eyelid muscles, wanting to eat again about an hour after an evening meal, no desire for breakfast, lapses in concentration, tenderness over the pancreas and sore trigger points over the left lower ribs.

## Other Conditions Associated with Unstable Blood Sugar Levels

While many doctors believe that low blood sugar levels are just something you get if you read too many women's magazines, others take the condition very seriously, believing that there is a connection between long-term hypoglycaemia and the development of chronic problems such as:

overweight
hyperactivity
anxiety
depression
asthma
loss of interest in sex
fainting
blackouts
facial pain
epilepsy
arthritis
allergies
migraine

stomach ulcers
addictions
tinnitus.

# PRINCIPLES OF EATING TO KEEP THE BLOOD SUGAR STABLE

## Hunger

The first rule is never to allow yourself to become hungry. The brain responds to the message of hunger by releasing adrenalin to access the store of sugar in the liver. High adrenalin levels produce trembling, headaches and the symptoms which have already been discussed.

## Dangers of Modern Eating Habits

Saving calories until the evening meal and having a 'blow out', perhaps because of fear of becoming overweight, is harmful in several ways.

- Fuel is needed during the day when you are active and less in the evening when you are resting.
- If the blood sugar levels are unstable during the day, by the time the pancreas is presented with the evening meal it is already so jittery that it may overcompensate with too much insulin and therefore within an hour or a little more after the meal your blood sugar level can be *lower than before you ate!* This is the time when you reach for biscuits, etc. You will probably have already done this mid-morning and mid-afternoon.

## Will I Gain Weight on a Diet to Stabilize Blood Sugar Levels?

You should *lose* weight, for three reasons:

1. Insulin is often called the fat hormone. The more insulin you produce the more fat you are likely to lay down.
2. You will not be consuming the 'empty', that is non-nutritious, calories of sugar and refined carbohydrates. These are the danger foods as far as excess weight is concerned.
3. Your energy levels should rise considerably. This will make you more active and you should metabolize your food more efficiently.

## What If I Lose Too Much Weight?

Simply increase the amount of complex carbohydrate, including potatoes, that you eat until your weight stabilizes. Also eat larger portions of allowed foods. Do not be tempted to revert completely to a high sugar diet, but perhaps you can be a little more flexible with dessert after your main meals.

## What Should I Eat?

### Carbohydrate

There are several approaches to eating plans to stabilize blood sugar levels. The one suggested is the most popular one. High whole-grain diets with or without meat, and the macrobiotic diet (see Kushi, Mishio, *Diabetes and Hypoglycaemia: A Natural Approach*, Japan Publications, 1985) can also be used.

Another approach is to restrict carbohydrate to two or three slices of wholemeal bread, or less, or the equivalent in crispbread such as Ryvita. Some of this ration could be eaten as a whole-grain cereal, for example porridge, for breakfast (add seeds or nuts). If you work hard physically you might need a little more. If you are sedentary and overweight you could probably manage on less. Many people panic at the thought of restricting carbohydrate. This is a very useful eating plan for the very obese or those who have difficulty digesting grains. There is no need to. If you are eating plenty of the allowed foods you should not be hungry.

## Vegetables

Eat as many as you wish, raw or cooked.

## Fruit

Include fresh fruit and unsweetened fruit juice to the equivalent of four to five pieces of fruit per day. This might seem more than what is allowed in other low blood sugar diets but should not be a problem unless you need to lose a lot of weight. The sugar in fruit (fructose) does not need insulin for digestion and therefore should not overstimulate the pancreas. The fruit and juice intake should include a high quantity of apple. Apple pectin helps to stabilize blood sugar levels.[2] Bananas are higher in carbohydrate than other fruits and should be limited to one per day.

## Protein

Many of the earlier hypoglycaemic diets were very high in protein, but this has been found to be unnecessary; normal helpings of animal or vegetable protein suffice. Protein is a vital part of this eating plan. If you do not eat protein with each main meal you will not stabilize your blood sugar levels and are much more likely to crave sweet foods.

## Fat

Unless you have been advised by your doctor to eat a low fat diet, include a moderate amount of fat in the diet. The trend for very low fat diets could have contributed to the rise in hypoglycaemia. There are also other hazards. Women on low fat diets have been shown to have a higher incidence of depression and suicidal tendencies.[3] A meal which includes fat stays much longer in the stomach than a low fat meal. Some of the foods you will be including actually reduce the cholesterol levels. They include apples, onions, garlic, olive oil and unrefined oats. Oat bran also has the advantage of stabilizing blood sugar levels.[4]

# Do Not Eat

## Refined Carbohydrates

All white flour products such as bread, biscuits, cakes, sweetened refined breakfast cereals and pastries are out.

## Sugar

Sugar in all forms, confectionery, dried fruit, soft drinks, is out. Look for hidden sugar in any prepared foods. In fact anything that tastes sweet, unless it states it contains only artificial sweeteners. These can be taken in small quantities, particularly at first if you are craving sugar. Liberal use helps to prolong your desire for sweet foods. If you keep to a sensible eating plan any desire for sweet foods should go within a few weeks.

# Suggested Diet

| | |
|---|---|
| *On waking* | small glass of unsweetened juice or a piece of fruit |
| *Breakfast* | more fruit juice |
| | *Cooked breakfast*: grilled bacon, fish, eggs, baked beans, sausages, nutburger, vegetarian sausage or any protein dish, *plus* mushrooms or tomatoes or any vegetable |

*Carbohydrate ration* (unless you have had porridge): one slice of whole-meal bread, two crispbreads, rice cakes, etc., with butter, margarine, nut butter, cottage cheese or cream cheese

OR

*Cold breakfast*: whole-oat porridge with a little salt and preferably some whole or ground nuts or seeds – or sweetened with a few sultanas, apple juice or artificial sweetener; or muesli made from whole oats, nuts, seeds (pumpkin, sunflower, etc.); or plain yogurt with fresh fruit and nuts, fruit yogurt, fromage frais, cottage cheese, cold ham or other meat, cheese

*Carbohydrate ration* (unless you have had porridge): as above

*Drinks*: weak tea with milk if desired, decaffeinated coffee, herb tea, milk

*No More than Two Hours after Breakfast*

*Snack*: fruit, apple and cheese, yogurt, milk, seeds, nuts, plus allowed drink

*Lunch*

any protein dish, hot or cold: meat, fish, cheese, eggs, chicken, sardines, tuna, pilchards, etc., or any bean, lentil or nut dish

|  | *Plus as much salad or as many cooked vegetables as you can eat* |
|---|---|
|  | *Carbohydrate ration* (unless you have had potatoes with your meal): 1 slice of wholemeal bread or 2 crispbreads |
| *Two and a Half to Three Hours after Lunch* | weak tea, herb tea, milk with crispbread, cheese, low-sugar jam, or the same as mid-morning break; this is often the time chosen to eat the daily banana |
| *Half an hour before dinner* | small glass of fruit juice |
| *Dinner* | same as lunch, plus fruit |
| *Supper* | crispbreads, butter, cheese, meat or fish paste, slice of cold meat, chicken and so on |
| *Drinks* | milk drink, weak tea, herb tea |

This might look like a lot of food, but remember there is no need to eat large quantities. Small and often is the rule.

## Quick Reference

- Don't skip meals.
- Eat the allowed foods at regular intervals.
- Always have protein in your meals, particularly breakfast.
- Make the overnight fast as short as possible; if you wake in the night have a snack containing protein or complex carbohydrate.
- Cut down or abstain from caffeine,[5] alcohol, cigarettes and street drugs.

- Never smoke or drink alcohol before a meal.
- Do not drink alcohol during the day.[6]
- Consider whether you are using too many 'over-the-counter' drugs.
- Check with your doctor to see if all the medication you are taking is necessary.
- Watch your stress levels.
- Adopt better breathing habits.
- Take graduated exercise.
- Avoid too many late nights.
- Take a course of the recommended supplements (unless this conflicts with advice from your doctor).
- Always carry a snack (seeds, nuts, fruit, whole-grain low-sugar bar) with you in case you get delayed.
- In an emergency buy potato crisps; if you can only find a chocolate bar choose one with nuts in it and follow it with a protein meal as soon as you can.
- Don't try to fit your eating plan around others – your diet is important, it is your medicine!

## Hypoglycaemia and Nutritional Supplements

### Chromium

Chromium is the keystone for the glucose tolerance factor known as GTF which is thought to play a central role in the balance of blood sugar levels. Even with a sensible diet it is difficult to get the 125 micrograms of daily chromium recommended.[7] Inorganic chromium is poorly absorbed; organic Bio-Chromium is available in health stores and should be taken as directed by the manufacturers or your practitioner. Some people feel better within a few weeks of starting supplementation but a course of three months is recommended.

## *Magnesium*

In an experimental controlled study of magnesium supplementation, blood glucose of hypoglycaemics failed to drop below fasting levels during glucose-tolerance tests; 57 per cent felt better versus 25 per cent of subjects on placebo.[8]

A six-week trial of around 340 mg daily for six weeks is suggested, unless you develop diarrhoea with this dose. Magnesium acts as a laxative.

People who have had nutritionally unsound diets for some time or those who are run-down could also include the supplements suggested for alcohol withdrawal below.


# ALCOHOL

The strong connection between hypoglycaemia and problem drinking cannot be denied. There is a wealth of scientific information on this subject. The symptoms of a hangover are, after all, hypoglycaemic symptoms. The person with an inherited tendency to hypoglycaemia is much more likely to have problems with alcohol for two reasons:

- The alcohol gives him/her the same fix as a high-sugar/junk-food diet.
- Alcohol makes the store of glucose in the liver less accessible and so the problem drinker is in a vicious circle. In reaching for alcohol to stop withdrawal symptoms (including those of hypoglycaemia) he/she is in turn reducing the supply of glucose which would help the symptoms. People with alcohol problems invariably have a history and/or family history of blood-sugar-related conditions, such as overweight, migraine, arthritis and so on.

The problem drinker is so often seen as a weak person who cannot cope with the problems of life, or is judged as being irresponsible and hedonistic. The fact is that alcohol craving can be the result of biochemical imbalances and, in spite of the enormous amount of research which supports this, it is usually disregarded in general medicine. Old-fashioned notions of pleasure-seeking behaviour and the need to apportion blame abound. Animal studies are interesting and show that alcohol craving has its origins in the body, particularly the brain, and not in the psyche.

Laboratory rats were divided into two groups. One group was provided with a high carbohydrate 'junk' diet, the other with a biologically ideal diet. Both groups were given a choice of water or alcohol to drink. Both groups with a high sugar diet turned to the alcohol for drink, while their better-fed neighbours drank only water. These animals were not under stress, resentful, depressed, unhappy or frustrated. They just turned willingly to alcohol when their diet was inadequate. Furthermore, they became reformed alcoholics when their diets were improved and their carbohydrate level reduced.[9]

## Giving Up or Cutting Down on Alcohol

What you do about your alcohol consumption will probably depend on the degree of your symptoms. When people fully understand what alcohol is doing to their blood sugar levels many are willing to abstain completely for a while. From others the cry is 'But does that mean I can never enjoy a drink again?' The answer is no. When the body is balanced and healthy it can stand the strain of moderate weekend drinking or a couple of glasses of wine with a meal. When the blood sugar levels are swinging and the nervous system is overstimulated even half a pint of lager can cause severe symptoms. Alcohol affects more than the blood sugar levels, and if you normally drink heavily it would certainly make sense to give your body a complete rest from it for about six months. If you have tried this before and it was hell, remember that you have more information now, and with the correct diet and supplements it should be a great deal easier. In fact a great many people have said they did not intend giving up drinking completely but the desire just went once they were established on the diet. Smokers will find the craving for nicotine diminishes too.

## Giving Up

- Do not attempt this until you have been on the diet or diet/supplements for at least four weeks, but if you could cut down to a level where you are still comfortable, do.
- After four weeks keep very strictly to the diet: eat as many raw vegetables and salads* as you can, and if necessary increase fruit and have drink diluted with apple juice when you would normally drink alcohol.
- Do not be tempted to increase your tea, coffee, coke intake.†
- Take gentle exercise and get as much rest as possible.
- Encourage detoxification.

---

* In an experimental study thirty-two hypertensive patients ate 62 per cent of their calories as raw food for six months; 80 per cent of those who smoked or drank abstained spontaneously.[10]

† In an animal experimental study[11] one group of rats was fed a junk-food diet, the other received a well-balanced nutritious diet. When given either caffeine or coffee *both* groups increased their alcohol intake. This is not surprising, since the caffeine would stimulate the production of insulin and the resultant hypoglycaemia would, in turn, make the rats turn to alcohol for their sugar fix.

## Gradual Withdrawal

- Start the diet and cut down to a third of your daily intake of alcohol.
- After four weeks cut down to one or two glasses of wine, a pint of beer or one measure of spirits daily in the evening.
- Exercise and encourage detoxification as above.

It might seem strange in the light of the earlier information on the vicious circle of alcohol and hypoglycaemia that immediate and complete abstinence is not recommended for all sufferers. The reason for this is that complete withdrawal can be an enormous strain; withdrawal symptoms, in addition to the headaches, panic attacks and so on that the severely hypoglycaemic person is already experiencing, would for some people be rather a lot to cope with. But in saying that, if you know you cannot open a bottle without finishing it, you would be foolish not to go for complete abstinence. Take heart, the end results will be well worth it.

# Alcohol/Hypoglycaemia and Behaviour

Hypoglycaemia is taken much more seriously in America as a cause of ill health and behavioural problems than it is in the United Kingdom. Studies have shown violent offenders in institutions to be happier and less aggressive when given a nutritional regime designed to keep blood sugar levels stable. The treatment has also been used for drunken drivers ('A diet for drunken drivers', *San Jose Mercury News*, 7 December 1993):

Jail time for some drunken drivers hasn't stopped them from again drinking and driving. Now, San Mateo County is trying a new approach – taking away their coffee and candy bars.

In what could become a model for the state, thirty convicted drunken drivers . . . will participate in a new programme aimed at curbing alcohol abuse.

The regimen? Eat three protein-rich meals a day – and reduce caffeine and sugar.

## Nutritional Supplements

There are three reasons why the long-term heavy drinker has many nutritional deficiencies: (1) alcohol inhibits absorption of essential vitamins and minerals; (2) the heavy drinker would rather drink than eat; and (3) the hypoglycaemia hangover prevents eating breakfast and often lunch, and high carbohydrate foods are craved towards evening.

Supplements and a well-balanced diet not only correct the nutritional status, but *can also do a great deal to minimize withdrawal symptoms and prevent relapse*. If possible, see a doctor who specializes in nutritional medicine, a nutritionist. (For telephone counselling see 'Useful Addresses': Nutrition Line.) There are also many alternative practitioners who are very knowledgeable on nutrition. Here are some suggestions for supplements you will find in your pharmacy or health food store.

CAUTION. Don't think that because you are swallowing a few supplements you can be careless about your eating habits. A well-balanced diet must be the choice if your income will not stretch to cover both.

### Vitamin B Complex

Choose a yeast-free one with 50 mg of the main Bs. People coming off alcohol are often prone to fungal infections (see Shirley Trickett, *Coping with Candida*). Headache sufferers often have a reaction to niacin B[3] (a harmless flushing and prickling of the skin which usually subsides within half an hour) so look for a product containing another form of B³ called nicotinamide. This has the same beneficial effect. B complex will make your urine a strange colour but don't let this cause you concern. The B vitamins can be stimulating, so take these with your breakfast. If you cannot tolerate the full dose build it up slowly by taking it three times a week or taking part of the tablet daily.

## Multi-mineral Tablet

This should include: calcium, magnesium, selenium, zinc and chromium (see p. 140).

## Evening Primrose Oil

This is an EFA or essential fatty acid; ½–1 g three times daily has been suggested to reduce the symptoms of alcohol withdrawal.[12] Some people get headaches when taking evening primrose oil. If you cannot tolerate it, fish oil capsules would also be helpful.

## Vitamin C

You can buy this in powder form from your pharmacist. It helps to rid the body of the toxins from the alcohol. This is another vitamin that can stimulate, so take it early in the day. If you can build up to 3 g per day without getting 'wired' – over-stimulated – or having digestive upsets it can be very beneficial.

CAUTION. Supplements should be regarded as a medicine and as such kept out of reach of children. They should be taken as a course until you are well and not, unless under medical supervision, as a lifelong medication.

# OTHER CAUSES OF BLOOD SUGAR PROBLEMS

## Caffeine

Caffeine is a powerful stimulant; it can be consumed in large quantities in coffee itself, and in tea, coke, chocolate and some headache medications. Caffeine pushes the adrenal glands to raise the blood sugar level and insulin levels have to increase to keep pace with this. It has a similar effect to sugar and in addition has addictive properties. When the blood sugar levels are severely disturbed a cup of coffee or strong tea could be enough to produce severe anxiety symptoms. When treating hypoglycaemia, it is wise to give up coffee (you won't be having coke or chocolate because of their sugar content), but a word of warning about withdrawal. Like any other drug some people are more affected by withdrawal than others. This depends on what is going on biochemically and is not just the longing for the taste of coffee. When some coffee drinkers (even people who just have one cup per day) abstain they can for a few days suffer severe headaches and nausea, and can feel depressed for a couple of weeks. This is really due to caffeine poisoning, known as the 'caffeine storm'. In the absence of ingested caffeine, the caffeine in the body is mobilized and causes problems until detoxification is complete. To avoid this, cut down slowly by mixing half of your regular coffee with decaffeinated and progress slowly until you are drinking all decaffeinated.

## Cigarettes

Nicotine stimulates the adrenal glands to release glucose into the blood. This is why it acts as an appetite suppressant. Your desire for nicotine should decrease when you are established on the hypoglycaemic eating plan.

## Prescribed Drugs and Blood Sugar Problems

If change of diet is the prime cause of low blood sugar problems in modern man, then the massive increase in the use of prescribed drugs must be the second. Medical evidence now clearly states that the contraceptive pill, steroids, tranquillizers and sleeping pills, beta blockers and some diuretics (water pills) affect glucose tolerance, cholesterol and triglyceride metabolism. This adverse reaction often goes unnoticed because it is not dramatic. The onset is insidious and often not associated with the drugs either by the doctor or the patient.[13] For information on how to withdraw safely from tranquillizers and sleeping pills see Shirley Trickett, *Coming off Tranquillisers and Sleeping Pills* (Thorsons).

## Non-prescribed Drugs

Street drugs, including heroin, cocaine and cannabis, all affect blood sugar levels and so when withdrawing from them the same principles of diet and nutritional supplementation apply as for alcohol withdrawal (above).

# CHILDREN AND HYPOGLYCAEMIA

The behaviour of pale, irritable children crying for sweets at the supermarket checkout after school is the responsibility of the parent, not the child. If the child was given a wholemeal sandwich or an apple and cheese as it came out of the school gates many of these scenes would not occur. Children expend a vast amount of energy at school and many do not have a sufficient food intake to keep their blood sugar levels stable until they get home for tea. Ensure:

- that your child has a protein breakfast;
- that you ask staff about the quantity of food the young child eats at lunchtime;
- that you provide bananas or an apple for mid-morning and mid-afternoon breaks;
- that you meet the child with a snack;
- that you provide a substantial snack for the older child who has activities such as swimming or dancing after school;
- that you don't make young children wait for a family meal at 6 p.m. or later; give them a meal earlier and a snack before bed.

Hypoglycaemic children are fretful children who sleep badly and succumb to infections readily. They are also more likely to suffer from frequent headaches, transient abdominal pain, tantrums, asthma, eczema, allergies and hyperactivity.

# CASE HISTORIES

I have written books on a variety of health problems and they all include a chapter on hypoglycaemia. I can justify this by the wonderful letters I get from people all over the world who say that simply by changing their eating habits they have changed their lives.

## Woman of Forty-seven

I read the literature on hypoglycaemia and in spite of several family members having conditions which would put me in line for hypoglycaemia I still did not take it seriously – it all seemed too simple. I had been a headache sufferer for years and often had palpitations and cold sweats. The doctor said it was my nerves. It was the accidental changing of my eating habits that made me take a second look at the information.

I was sent on a residential course for a week. Because they were put in front of me I ate three meals a day. I had not eaten a cooked breakfast for years. It was a boring week but I did notice that I had more energy and slept better. I thought it was just the change of scene.

On return home I reverted to my usual eating pattern and was rewarded with my familiar symptoms!

I have kept strictly to the diet now for seven months and feel a different person. I put on six pounds at first but am now back to my normal weight.

## Woman of Thirty-nine

I had high levels of sugar in my urine when carrying my first child (my grandmother was diabetic and my mother asthmatic). I was given a series of glucose tolerance tests, all of which gave me severe headaches and the shakes. My husband said it was the fear of the needles that made me nervous but I knew it was not that. I have never been afraid of injections. (He is the one with the needle phobia!) I was diagnosed as pre-diabetic and told to keep my weight down to avoid maturity-onset diabetes. That was all the information I was given. The result was that for years I ate very little all day and had a big evening meal. I had years of being very uncomfortable after this meal; restlessness, palpitations, hot and cold flushes, and sometimes an inexplicable feeling of doom. I also had difficulty getting off to sleep and would wake regularly at 3.20 a.m. I knew the symptoms were something to do with eating, so I suspected food allergies.

This was the wrong path and I was as frustrated as ever when I tried elimination diets.

I became a frequent user of the health section in the library and it was there I found a book on panic attacks which mentioned hypoglycaemia − it was all there. I feel a totally different person since I have been on the diet and know when I have 'lapsed'. I usually pay the penalty the next day in the form of a headache or a hung-over feeling.

## REFERENCES

1. Davies, Stephen, and Stewart, Alan, *Nutritional Medicine*, Pan Books, 1987

2. Werbach, Melvyn R., *Nutritional Influences on Illness: A Sourcebook of Clinical Research*, Thorsons, 1987

3. Hyman, Engelberg, 'Low-serum cholesterol and suicide', *Lancet*, 339 (21 March 1992), 727

4. Werbach, op. cit.

5. Ashton, C. H., 'Caffeine and health', *British Medical Journal*, 295, 6609 (21 November 1987), 1293

6. O'Keefe, S.J.D., and Marks, V., 'Lunchtime gin and tonic as a cause of reactive hypoglycaemia', *Lancet*, 1 (1977), 1286

7. *North East Times* (September 1989)

8. ibid.

9. Budd, Martin L., *Low Blood Sugar (Hypoglycaemia): The Twentieth-century Epidemic?*, Thorsons, 1981

10. Werbach, op.cit.

11. Register, O., et al., *Journal of the American Dietetics Association*, 61 (1972), 159–62

12. Horrobin, D. F., ed., *Clinical Uses of Essential Fatty Acids*, Eden Press, 1982

13. Taylor, Ron, 'Drugs and glucose tolerance', *Adverse Drug Reaction Bulletin*, (Newcastle Health Authority), 121 (December 1986)

## FURTHER READING

Trickett, Shirley, *Recipes for Health: Candida Albicans*, Thorsons, 1995
   Although the recipes in this book are designed to discourage fungal overgrowth in the bowel, since they are sugar-free and low in carbohydrate they are equally useful for controlling low blood sugar problems. They are designed to fit in with family meals.

# 11

# Headaches and Changing Hormone Levels

Headaches frequently accompany the changing hormone levels of puberty, the premenstrual phase, the menopause and pregnancy, although in pregnancy, particularly in the later stages (possibly because hypoglycaemia is less likely at this time), a woman may for a time be relieved of the migrainous headaches she has suffered from for years.

## HEADACHES IN THE PREMENSTRUAL AND MENSTRUAL PHASE

These fall into three groups:

- those caused by swollen cells; they are characterized by constant pain in the cheek-bones and forehead extending over to the back of the head, and sometimes accompanied by a stuffy nose and difficult breathing;
- tension headaches caused by the effect of changing hormone levels on mood;
- migraines caused by hormonal influences on the blood vessels in the brain.

## The Premenstrual Phase

This can be described as a set of symptoms which appears seven to ten days before menstruation and disappears during or after menstruation. For some women it is just a minor cyclical discomfort. For others, it is a dreaded, fearful illness which destroys their confidence in themselves and their fitness for motherhood, and often their relationships with their partners and their ability to hold down a job. The symptoms are due to physiological changes which include changes in brain chemistry; the sufferers are perfectly well at other times in the month and are not 'neurotic' or hysterical, as sadly they are often labelled. The symptoms include:

fatigue
headaches
palpitations
dizziness or fainting
constipation
fluid retention
swollen abdomen, thighs, ankles, hands and face
tender breasts
tingling of the fingers (usually the little and adjacent finger)
numbness in the hands and arms after sleeping
clumsiness – particularly dropping things
low backache
muscle and joint pains
disturbance of blood sugar levels
food cravings, extreme hunger
temporary food intolerance
restlessness
irritability
hopelessness

insomnia

anxiety, phobias, panic attacks, depersonalization

depression

mood swings

violent feelings, actual violence

suicidal feelings, suicide attempts

oily skin or acne

Women who have conditions such as asthma often have a worsening of symptoms premenstrually.[1] This is not surprising, since asthma can be affected by changing blood sugar levels.

## Regular Comments from Sufferers

'I am a totally different person one week in four.'

'Each time, I think I'm going mad.'

'I can't convince my doctor about how ill I feel. He just offers me antidepressants.'

'It's the only time I ever smack the children. The guilt destroys me.'

'I know I will lose my husband if I don't get some help.'

'I'm terrified by how aggressive I feel – it's just not me. I never feel like that at any other time.'

'I have to get my mother to come to stay every month. I'm so afraid I will do something stupid. I don't feel like this at any other time. She was frightened at first but now she understands.'

'I live in terror of my children being taken into care. During that week they are strangers to me. My husband says I'm just being ridiculous.'

'I feel like a lumbering elephant and keep bumping into things.'

'My whole body aches as if I had flu.'

'As soon as I start to pass more urine the relief is immediate; my mood lifts.'

'I feel as if my head is bursting before my period.'

## What To Do about PMT

- Look carefully at your diet. How does it differ from the suggested diet for low blood sugar problems?
- How much exercise are you getting? You must move if you want the lymphatic system to work properly. Brisk daily walking for half an hour *during the whole of the month* should help to prevent retention of fluid. A weekly workout or aerobics class is not enough – a helpful extra, but not enough in itself.
- Look at your lifestyle. Look ahead to the end of the month and plan to take it easier during that time.
- Bombard your partner with literature on PMT.
- Explain to the children *before* the event that sometimes you feel irritable and that it is not their fault. Appeal to them to help you on the days when you are feeling unwell. Get them to colour on the calendar the days when you know your fuse will be short.
- If there is any extra help around, ask for it. You cannot help being subject to your hormones.
- Don't be ashamed of how you feel – unless of course you are not willing to look at how you can help yourself.

## Nutritional Supplements and PMT

Many sufferers find that adjusting the diet and taking supplements either completely cures or alleviates their symptoms. There are sound physiological reasons for this.

### Magnesium

Magnesium has been shown to increase progesterone levels in the premenstrual phase[2] and also reduces the symptoms of reactive hypoglycaemia (low blood sugar), which for many women is a large part of the PMT syndrome.

## Vitamin B6

This vitamin increases red-cell magnesium levels and also helps to prevent fluid retention. Prescribed diuretics often deplete magnesium levels and therefore compound the problem.[3]

## Vitamin B Complex

The B vitamins should never be taken in isolation because they deplete the store of the other B vitamins. So if you are taking vitamin B6, it is necessary to take a small dose of B complex daily or a larger dose two or three times a week. During the pre-menstrual phase 100 mg B6 is necessary daily; 50 mg or less can be taken during the rest of the month. Some people find B complex gives them headaches. If this is your experience include as many foods rich in vitamin B in your diet as possible.

## Essential Fatty Acids

We need fat in various forms to maintain health, including lino-leic and linolenic acids – the 'essential fatty acids'. They have to be taken in the diet because they cannot be manufactured by the body. Foods high in EFAs include sunflower seeds, fish, shellfish, fish liver oils, safflower seed oil, corn oil, lean meat, kidneys, liver, pulses and green vegetables. Evening primrose oil is a very rich source. Your doctor may prescribe this for PMT. Vitamins B6 and C, and zinc are necessary for the absorption of evening prim-rose oil. A combination of these, called Efamol, is available at most pharmacies. Some people are unable to utilize their dietary intake of EFAs and research has shown that many conditions such as PMT, cardiovascular problems, rheumatoid arthritis, eczema, hyperactivity in children, inflammatory conditions, dry eye and even multiple sclerosis and schizophrenia can be helped by supplementation. For more information on this see Judy Graham's *Evening Primrose Oil: Its Remarkable Properties and Its Use in the Treatment of a Wide Range of Conditions* (Thorsons, 1984).

If you want more information ring Nutrition Line (see Useful Addresses) or The Premenstrual Advisory Service, Box 268, Hove, Sussex: tel. 01273 771366.

# THE CONTRACEPTIVE PILL

If you feel the pill is giving you headaches read Ellen Grant's *The Bitter Pill – How Safe is the 'Perfect Contraceptive'?* (Elm Tree Books, 1985).

# HORMONE REPLACEMENT THERAPY

Some women feel wonderful on HRT, others suffer headaches and feel bloated and depressed. A natural HRT treatment is boron, a substance found in green vegetables. Clinical trials have found this supplement (often combined with calcium) as useful as synthetic hormones for controlling menopausal symptoms. It is available in most health stores or from Nutrition Line. This organization can also give you details of an exciting new cream called Pro-gest, which is used for menopausal problems, including osteoporosis. It is made from wild yams. Many doctors are prescribing this and the results are impressive.

## REFERENCES

1. Davies, Stephen, and Stewart, Alan, *Nutritional Medicine: The Drug-free Guide to Better Family Health*, Pan Books, 1987
2. ibid.
3. Trimmer, Eric, *The Magic of Magnesium*, Thorsons, 1987

## BIBLIOGRAPHY

Davies, Stephen, 'Magnesium in health, disease and practice', *Journal of Alternative Medicine*, December 1983, p. 17

# 12

# Headaches and Other Problems Caused by Hyperventilation

I have covered this subject more fully in my book *Coping Successfully with Panic Attacks*. If any of the books mentioned are not in your local library, they will order them for you for a small charge.

Six to eleven per cent of patients seen in a doctor's surgery breathe in a manner that causes health problems. The symptoms produced are often misdiagnosed because most doctors only recognize the symptoms of overt hyperventilation and overlook the signs of chronic subtle hyperventilation (overbreathing).

In common with hypoglycaemia, hyperventilation (sometimes called collar-bone breathing) is often seen simply as a sign of anxiety. Overt hyperventilation, where the patient is panting, gasping for breath and in an agitated state, is well recognized, but chronic low-grade hyperventilation is often not immediately obvious. The chronic hyperventilator breathes shallowly and rapidly, usually more than sixteen times per minute, using only the upper part of the chest. The breaths often vary in depth, with an occasional deep, sighing breath. Breathing in this way deprives the brain of carbon dioxide. Any experienced telephone counsellor will be familiar with this sound. This breathing contrasts with normal breathing, which uses the abdominal muscles and where there is very little upper chest movement; it is silent and gentle, with a resting breathing rate of about eight to twelve breaths per minute.

It is unlikely that headaches will be the symptom of hyperventilation that takes you to the doctor, because the headaches are not usually severe – rather more generalized, dull headaches with a 'spacy' feeling. If you are overbreathing to the extent of getting very tense, you may have tension headaches. Migraine can also be triggered by hyperventilation.[1]

## First Aid for Symptoms of Hyperventilation

To re-breathe the carbon dioxide you are losing, place a paper bag around the nose and mouth, drop your shoulders and relax in a chair or on the bed. If you puff and blow into the bag you will make the symptoms worse. Just sit there and imagine your breathing becoming slower and slower. Continue for at least ten minutes and, if possible, have a rest or relax with a book afterwards. Do this as many times as you wish during the day or night.

## Why Do People Develop This Breathing Habit?

Hyperventilation is another mechanism which suppresses feeling. It acts in the same way as the tightening of the muscles – it keeps in our emotions. Stress is the major cause of hyperventilation; some others follow.

### Emotional Triggers

These include suppression of fear, sadness, grief, anger and frustration.

It is natural for the breathing rate to increase when we are in a fearful situation. This gives us the impetus to run or challenge. When we are in a chronically anxious state we are continually halfway to the emergency mode and our breathing matches that state. Breath-holding can be a feature of hyperventilation. This could be an unconscious attempt to slow down the metabolism and the overproduction of adrenalin.

### Physical Triggers

The only positive thing which can be said about hyperventilation (unless we are in a flight-or-fight situation) is that it can help to control physical pain, particularly in the chest and back. Imagine breathing deeply with broken ribs. The danger lies in the fact that often long after the pain has gone the sufferer retains the habit of overbreathing.

Tight clothing, working for long periods in a cramped position, gas in the stomach or bowel pushing up on the diaphragm, a stuffy nose, excitement, compulsive talking or muscular tension can all cause overbreathing. It could also be that deficiency of the B vitamins and a poor nutritional state could be another factor. A high-sugar diet can also be a cause, so the symptoms of hypoglycaemia and hyperventilation can coexist.

Taking a deep breath after relaxing may be an unconscious trigger which starts a hyperventilation attack. For this reason I am wary of commercial relaxation tapes which instruct people to take deep breaths.

## How Does the Body Respond to Hyperventilation?

When the full capacity of the lungs is not utilized the correct balance of oxygen and carbon dioxide in the blood cannot be maintained, and the result is an alteration in brain chemistry which can lead to uncomfortable and often bizarre symptoms.

Even if carbon dioxide levels do not fall enough to give rise to dramatic neurological symptoms, continually overbreathing can result in being continually tired and in a nervous state. Because the onset of these symptoms is insidious and the sufferer may have had them for many years, it is often difficult to convince the person with poor breathing habits that they are themselves creating the symptoms which are disrupting their lives. Just as in hypoglycaemia, where sudden changes in blood sugar levels can cause dramatic symptoms, with hyperventilation sudden changes in carbon dioxide levels can produce dizziness, panic and headaches. This is why some people are so afraid to let go in a relaxation class; a few deep breaths can rapidly give rise to symptoms.

## Symptoms of Overbreathing

Yawning (air hunger)
Light-headedness
Dizziness
Headaches and migraine
Anxiety
Panic attacks
Depression
Feelings of unreality
Sense of hopelessness
Poor memory
Agoraphobia
Other phobias
Palpitations
Shortage of breath: inability to take deep breaths, frequent sighing (80 per cent of patients who hyperventilate sigh)
Dry throat: clearing of throat, moistening of dry lips
Dry cough: due to water and heat loss from mucosal lining of airway

Stuffy nose: dryness, sores in the nose, sniffing, dry lips

Chest pain: either a sharp pain lasting seconds or minutes or a dull ache over the heart and around the breastbone and ribs. This is caused by the strain on the muscles and ligaments by breathing continually from the upper chest.

Finger pressure around breastbone or ribs can often find very sore spots. There is also an inability to lie on the left side. The pain is not usually affected by breathing.

It can occur after exercise. Pressure from gas in the stomach can also cause pain.

Spasm in the coronary artery can cause severe pain and often people arrive at accident and emergency departments (sometimes several times a year) with this

Feeling of impending fainting: all ages

Actual fainting: more common in the young

Tingling: hands, feet and around mouth

Weakness: in all muscles

Numbness: anywhere in the body

Jelly legs: a feeling that the legs cannot support the body

Digestive disturbances: water brash, bloating, belching, wind in bowel, air swallowing, food intolerances, irritable bowel syndrome

Muscle spasm: particularly in the neck and shoulders; claw-like spasm in the hands and feet

Speech difficulties: feeling of tongue being swollen

Hallucinations: only when symptoms are severe. Children sometimes take gulping breaths and spin each other round in order to see 'pictures'

Increase in the effect of alcohol

Allergies: histamine production is increased by hyperventilation. Hyperventilators frequently exhibit food intolerances and have irritable bowel symptoms.[2]

CAUTION. Hyperventilation can mimic many organic diseases. Consult your doctor if you have any of the above symptoms. If he/she can find no organic cause for your symptoms (they are far more likely to say you have nervous trouble than to notice your breathing), don't worry – get started on the exercises given below.

Several factors foster the neglect of hyperventilation as a positive diagnosis, e.g. the absence of conspicuous overbreathing. Shortness of breath is seldom the primary complaint. But most important is the too-ready acceptance of the blanket diagnosis of 'neurosis' or 'anxiety state' to cover the inability of physicians to explain multiple symptoms without overt pathology.[3]

## Headaches and Hyperventilation

These are generalized, accompanied by a 'spacy' feeling and are not usually severe.

## How Do I Know If I am Hyperventilating?

If you have not identified with several of the symptoms in the above list your breathing patterns may not be a problem. For an additional check, count how many times you breathe per minute when you are at rest. If you feel anxious about this, however, your breathing will automatically speed up, so you might prefer to ask a friend to observe your breathing rate when you are not aware of what he/she is doing. The rise and fall of the chest count as one respiration. To calculate your breathing rate, look at a clock or watch with a second hand when you have been at rest for about ten minutes, count your respirations for thirty seconds and double this number; this will give you your breathing rate per minute. If it is sixteen or more you would be wise to start breathing retraining. Some people try to rush this and complain of feeling breathless and panicky. If you attempt to go from rapid shallow breathing to deep breaths you *will* feel odd. If you have been breathing rapidly and shallowly for years, then it is going to take time to correct this, but with patience, just as your present breathing pattern has become habit, so will the fuller, slower breaths which will nourish all the cells of your body and calm your nervous system.

## What to Do

Initially you should forget about how you are breathing and concentrate on expanding the chest cavity. If your shoulders are held high, and your ribs and abdomen tense, they must be constricting your lungs. You cannot expect your lungs to work efficiently under these conditions. It's rather like trying to inflate a balloon in a cereal box!

### The Muscles

1. Lie down or relax in a chair with your head supported.

2. Drop your shoulders.

3. Put your hands on your abdomen and push them up towards the ceiling with your abdomen – relax, and then repeat twice more. Think about the muscles, not your breathing, as you do this.

4. Place your hands, fingers pointing to the centre, on your ribs. Push the ribs out to the sides as far as you can. There should now be a gap between your hands. Relax and repeat twice.

5. Pull your shoulders up towards your ears and then release them and push your hands down your thighs as far as you can. Repeat twice more.

Do not rush any of these exercises. Relax as much as you need to between them. Notice the feelings in your shoulders after you have let them go and don't be surprised if your gut rumbles – it has just been released from prison.

## The Breath

As you move around in your normal activity, avoid holding your shoulders around your ears and attempt to slow down your breathing *gradually*; making the out-breath longer than the in-breath will be a good start – remember, at this stage it is slow breathing, not deep breathing, you are aiming for. If you can do the following exercise twice daily and be vigilant about slowing your breathing at all times, the old habits will gradually fade. Don't expect miracles overnight – it has taken time to establish your present breathing habits and it will take time to correct them.

## Relaxation Using the Complete Breath

1. Massage under the instep of each foot firmly in a circular motion (the reason for this will be explained in the section on 'grounding' on p. 196).

2. Lie down on the floor or bed with the head slightly raised. If you have back trouble, bend your knees and put your feet flat on the floor. If it is an effort to get up and down, relax in a chair with the head supported. Have a blanket near you. Initially relaxation can promote warmth but some people become very cold as deep tensions leave the body.

3. Choose a colour. Blue or green are the most sedating colours but you might prefer another. Imagine you are breathing this colour up through the soles of your feet and it is going to gently lift your abdomen, ease out your ribs, go up into your shoulders and neck and out of the top of your head. Let it then cascade like a glittering fountain down over your body

and over your feet. This must be done gently and rhythmically, like a slow wave washing up and over you.

4. Imagine the glow from this colour spreading to an area of about five feet around your body.

If you can, do this twice daily (on waking and before your evening meal, if possible) for ten minutes initially. Many people find the exercise boring and difficult at first but with patience you will soon enjoy the feeling so much that you want to extend the time – the longer you do it the more relaxed you will feel. Some people like to play music during their breathing exercises. If you get in a muddle just take a rest and start again.

## What Else Can I Do to Help My Breathing?

You can try graduated exercise, even simple stretching movements in the house, building up to brisk walking, swimming and, with your doctor's approval, aerobic exercise. Yoga is very helpful since it incorporates stretching and breathing exercises.

## Are There Breathing Retraining Clinics in the NHS?

There are a few hospitals where physiotherapists work with people to retrain their breathing, but unfortunately, unless you are severely agoraphobic or are overtly hyperventilating, it is unlikely that you would be referred.

## Alternative Therapies

Many alternative therapies can help hyperventilators. They include shiatsu, remedial massage and yoga.

## Excerpts from Sufferers' Letters

I endorse what you say about hyperventilation in your book on panic attacks. Several years ago I was severely agoraphobic and generally very nervous. After a six-week breathing retraining course at Papworth Hospital I felt like a completely new person. I continued the treatment at home and within four months was able to go alone to the local shops. I am now totally free of nervous troubles and travel all over.

I refused to believe I was overbreathing and that my breathing could have anything to do with how I felt until my therapist asked me to visualize driving over a bridge (my worst fear). As I did this, although I was not aware of my breathing speeding up, all the familiar feelings of panic, tingling fingers and dizziness came. I found the exercises a bit tedious at first and it took me several weeks to really let go but I have to admit I feel much more in control and I have lost all those strange physical feelings.

I have never had a panic attack but what I called my 'queer heads', shortness of breath and digestive problems have gone since I learned how to breathe from my abdomen.

## REFERENCES

1. Lumb, L. C., 'Hyperventilation syndromes in medicine and psychiatry: a review', *Journal of the Royal Society of Medicine*, 80 (April 1987), 229
2. ibid.
3. Lumb, L. C., 'Hyperventilation and anxiety state', *Journal of the Royal Society of Medicine*, 74 (January 1981)

# PART TWO

# Taking Care of Your General Health

# Paying Attention to General Health

## The Bowel

This might seem like an odd place to start when looking at measures to improve the general health. Perhaps most people would expect the accent to be on exercise and fresh air, with a footnote at the end reminding the reader to avoid constipation. When you understand that the bowel is not just a waste-disposal system but a vital part of your immune system, and learn how it plays a large part in determining your nutritional status, you might be more interested in learning how to keep it healthy.

A sluggish colon produces putrefaction. It was formerly thought that toxins from the colon could not enter the bloodstream; this is now known to be incorrect. Sufferers from the 'leaky gut syndrome' often get headaches.

## What is a Toxic Colon?

'Toxic colon' is the term for a bowel which is carrying old faeces. It is not only a major factor in the development of the irritable bowel syndrome, food intolerances and chronic vague ill health, but it can also cause degenerative disease such as arthritis and cancer. You cannot expect to be well if the main organ responsible for ridding the body of toxic waste is underfunctioning. When the colon is irritated by diet, stress, drugs, chemicals and so on, it tries to protect itself by producing more mucus; this can bind with the sludge from refined foods, such as white flour, and build up on the wall of the bowel and narrow the passage. This layer of gluey, hardened faeces (which can weigh 3–4 kg and accounts for many distended abdomens) is not only an excellent breeding ground for harmful organisms, but also prevents the production of enzymes necessary for digestion, inhibits the production of vitamins and hinders absorption of essential vitamins and minerals taken in the diet.

## Once a Day?

Do not think that, because you have regular bowel movements or even diarrhoea, you have escaped this problem. The stool can pass daily through a dirty colon and leave the accumulated residue on the walls behind. There is no need to get panicky about this, as there is a great deal that can be done about it.

## How Does a Toxic Colon Affect the Body?

The local effects of this poisonous residue are irritation and inflammation. The general effects include diarrhoea, constipation, fatigue, headaches, dull eyes, poor skin, spots, aching muscles, joint pains and depression. The poisons circulate via the blood through a network of vessels called the lymphatic system to all parts of the body. Healthy lymphatic fluid should serve to nourish cells not fed by blood vessels; the lymphatic fluid also kills off harmful organisms and carries away the refuse. If the body has to pump around excessive toxic waste long-term it is not surprising that it sometimes has to give up and the disease process takes over: irritable bowel syndrome, colitis (inflammation of the colon), Crohn's disease (inflammation of the small intestine), colon cancer and diverticulitis.

## Keeping the Colon Clean

The benefits of colon cleansing are manifold, not only in terms of health but also with regard to appearance: the skin looks vibrant, cellulite, water retention and blemishes disappear and the whites of the eyes regain a youthful clearness. How quickly you want to clean out is your choice.

## What to Do

Changing to a clean diet over a period of several weeks is described in my book *The Irritable Bowel Syndrome and Diverticulosis* (Thorsons). If you also want to lose weight, two books on clean eating with a common-sense approach are *The Wright Diet* by Celia Wright (Grafton, 1986) and *Fit for Life* by Harvey and Marilyn Diamond (Bantam, 1987).

*Cleansing the Colon* by Brian Wright (available from New Nutrition – see 'Useful Addresses') is an excellent booklet which describes how you can achieve a complete colon cleanse by diet, natural supplements and herbs.

## Colonic Irrigation

This practice had some bad press years ago because obsessive dieters abused it, but three or four treatments can be of tremendous value to remove an accumulation of old faeces. Most people think of this as some nightmare experience. It is far from this and there are many trained practitioners around the country using sterile up-to-date equipment. Some people feel lighter, and lose headaches, aches and pains, and other chronic symptoms after the first treatment. It is a swift method of cleansing the colon and it also obviates many of the unpleasant symptoms of detoxification. A sterile tube is inserted into the rectum and filtered water washes around the colon. It leaves via an evacuation tube, taking with it the accumulated debris and mucus of years. If you want to find a practitioner in your area write to the Colonic International Association, 16 Englands Lane, London NW3; tel. 0171 483 1595.

## The Spine

A rigid or stiff spine causes not only local pain but can also affect the internal organs. Osteopaths and chiropractors believe that a flexible, straight spine is essential for a healthy body. Slight displacements of the vertebrae (called subluxations) interfere with the nerve supply, cause the surrounding muscles to go into spasm and can also be the cause of organic problems. Subluxation in the mid-thoracic region will not only cause discomfort between the shoulders but can also be the cause of digestive problems. Problems with the cervical spine often cause headaches and migraine.

It is a strain for man to be upright all day and support the head, which comprises quite a large portion of the body weight. A few simple stretching exercises daily could save you a lot of back problems. Here are some suggested by Paul Lambeth, a shiatsu expert.

Another valuable ten minutes could be spent in the position taught in Alexander lessons, which allows the bones of the spine to fall into their natural positions and gives the muscles an opportunity to rest at their full length.

It is amazing how refreshed you feel after this short rest. Try to do it in the middle of the day. The office floor is as good as anywhere. Use telephone directories or paperback books – as many as will make up the width of your palm – to support your head. Don't forget to bend your knees, particularly if you suffer from back pain.

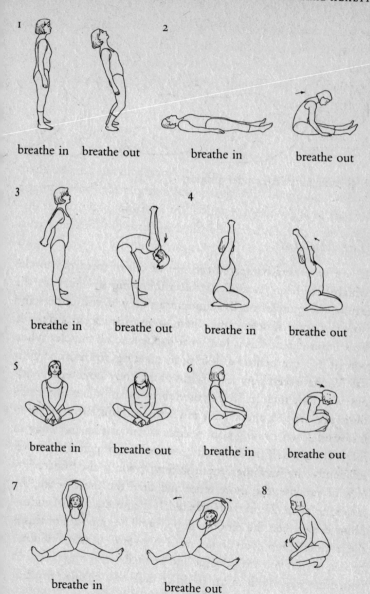

7. Shiatsu – controlled breathing ensures maximum stretch

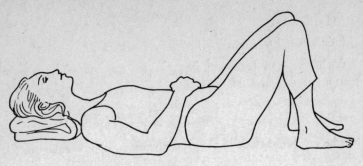

8. Resting in the Alexander position

## The Muscles

If you have ever compared the size of calf or forearm muscles which have been encased in plaster following an injury, to the size of the muscles on the uninjured side you will understand how not using muscles causes them to become flaccid and weak. To a lesser extent this is just what happens to all muscles when you sit in a car, behind a desk or in meetings for most of your day. We have seen how the systems of the body are interdependent: when the muscles are not used the waste products of metabolism are trapped, and aching and stiffness result; the circulation is slowed down, causing poor peripheral circulation and sluggish internal organs. If the lymphatic system cannot perform its task efficiently, the immune system suffers. Mood is also affected by lack of exercise: the more tense and tired the muscles are, the more the brain chemistry is affected. If the production of endorphins is low, then the mood will be low. The opposite of this is the 'runner's high'. You do not need to go as far as that, but don't be surprised if you are lethargic and mentally weary if you spend your time moving from car to office desk to a chair in front of the television set.

## How Much Do I Move My Body Each Day?

Even if you have little time for planned exercise, you can build simple stretching movements into your daily routine by stretching your calf muscles as you walk upstairs, avoiding lifts and escalators; taking a brisk walk in your lunch break; rotating your shoulders while waiting for the kettle to boil; making a habit of doing a few stretching exercises before your shower.

This might all sound very tame but at least it is a start; it might also make you aware of how much your body needs exercise. At least it is better than doing nothing and better than a frenetic visit to an exercise class which makes you stiff and sore and discourages you from going again.

## The Skin

Since it is the largest excretory organ of the body, encouraging detoxification by skin brushing or water therapies is an important part of getting fitter.

## Skin Brushing

If you brush all over with a dry skin brush (available from Boots and New Nutrition) for about ten minutes before your bath or shower you will greatly stimulate your circulation, help the release of toxins and improve the texture of your skin. Avoid tender or broken skin, moles and pimples. After a few days you will notice how the normally roughened areas such as knees, feet and elbows become smoother and softer.

# IMPROVING YOUR GENERAL HEALTH

## Water Therapies

The healing properties of water have been known for thousands of years. Even without considering it a therapy we would gravitate to a hot bath to relax tense muscles or to a cool shower to stimulate us if we were feeling listless and had a task to complete. Here are a few more suggestions about making the most of water.

## Cold Bathing

Although the benefits to the nervous system and circulation through the use of cold water have been recognized for centuries, only recently have scientists been able to use modern technology to discover what actually happens to the body when it is subjected to cold-water therapy. The treatment now known as thermo-regulatory hydrotherapy (TRHT) first hit the headlines about two years ago in a *European* supplement, 'An Amazing Discovery'. The coverage revealed that even before the newspaper had gone to press the message had flashed around the world – the paper had a medical scoop. The switchboard was flooded with calls from all over the world: Italian newspapers highlighted the hormonal effects of TRHT; *La Nazione* ran a headline 'More Sex with Cold Water'. The research is the work of Professor Vijay Kakkar of the Thrombosis Research Institute in London. TRHT boosts circulation, thereby increasing the amount of oxygen in body cells, leading to the improvement or cure of various conditions. According to Professor Kakkar these include circulatory problems, poor lymph drainage, asthma (from which he himself suffered), ME (the post-viral or chronic fatigue syndrome, myalgic encephalitis) and hormonal problems. As with any therapy there are health warnings. Here they are as they appeared in the *European*:

- Do not attempt THRT if you are suffering from well-established heart disease, high blood pressure or other chronic medical illnesses requiring medication, without first consulting your doctor.
- Do not be tempted to speed up the programme outlined by increasing the duration of therapy or suddenly lowering the temperature of the water recommended at each stage.
- THRT is not recommended for children below the age of thirteen. However, if practised, it must be under strict medical supervision.
- Do not smoke in the bath.
- Do not attempt to warm the body rapidly after the therapy by taking a hot bath or shower.
- The best way to get warm is to dress quickly, have a hot drink and eat something with enough carbohydrate in it to provide the energy required to meet the demand of increased metabolic activity.
- Do not undertake physical exercise after completing the THRT session. If you do wish to exercise, it is strongly advisable to do so before therapy.

## The Four Stages of the Therapy

Stage 1    Adaptation of the feet to cold water and touch
Stage 2    Adaptation of the lower half of the body in cold water
Stage 3    Total body immersion
Stage 4    Rewarming phase

The therapy takes thirty minutes per day and the water temperature is gradually lowered over a period of eighty days. For full instructions on THRT (article, temperature chart, bath thermometer) or if you wish to be a volunteer for this therapy contact: The Beatrice Hydrotherapy Centre, Sloane Square, London: tel. 0171 730 5319.

NOTE: Headache sufferers are welcomed for this treatment but not all migraine sufferers are found to be suitable and have to be seen by the physician first.

I can personally recommend this treatment although I have to admit I found it boring at first. After a few sessions I was willing to tolerate this for the wonderful feeling in my spine and muscles, which often lasted several hours. I felt the treatment relaxed me and increased my energy levels.

## Not So Drastic

If the idea of total immersion in cold water does not appeal, you can try foot baths and still gain some benefit. The skin of the feet has a large number of nerve endings. (A daily foot massage for about ten minutes can also be helpful. It helps the elimination of toxins and aids relaxation. When you first try this you will notice tender areas on the feet. As you continue to massage the tenderness decreases. You may feel hardness or grittiness in these areas, which you can disperse with continued massage.)

## 'Getting Cold Feet'

Stamping in cold water in the bath (for safety use a rubber bath mat) for three to five minutes or, better still, walking at the edge of the sea massages the soles of the feet and stimulates the hypothalamus gland. This increases the metabolic rate and produces a feeling of well-being.

## 'Getting into Hot Water'

The profuse sweating of a fever is nature's way of detoxifying the body. You can do this artificially in Turkish baths and saunas, or at home in salt or Epsom salts (magnesium) or seaweed baths.

These are all available from most pharmacists in large packs. A rough guide is to use about 2 lb of salt, 3 cups full of Epsom salts or one cupful of seaweed in a warm bath. The latter must be mixed to a paste in cold water and added gradually. Wrap up in a warm towel and rest for half an hour after your bath. Saunas and jacuzzis are also helpful for detoxification and relaxation.

## Swimming

Regular swimming can help your mind as well as your muscles, but remember that doing the breaststroke, particularly with your face out of the water, can cause tension in the neck and shoulder muscles and this often results in headaches, pain in the neck and shoulders, and also backache. Water exercises are just as useful as swimming: walking or jogging back and forth across the pool; rotating the shoulders backwards underwater; pushing the arms from side to side underwater or holding on to the side and working with one leg at a time, rotating ankle, knee and hip joints, and then kicking the leg as far forward and backward as possible.

## Fresh Air

Filling the lungs with clean air has a tonic effect on the whole body. At one time seeking fresh air was just a matter of being out of the house. Unfortunately in these polluted times we have to look actively for places where the air is fit to breathe. Make plans to be in the countryside or by the sea as much as possible, and during the week spend your lunch break in any green space, away from cars, that you can find; trees help to absorb pollution.

## Electrical Pollution

Emissions of smoke and fumes from industry and motor vehicles are well known to foul the air and most people avoid such polluted areas when they can. Less well known is the effect on human health of electrical pollution. Living or working near high-voltage electricity cables has been clearly shown to affect the immune system and cause depression. We also live and work in electrically polluted spaces – badly ventilated rooms filled with electrical equipment such as VDUs, television sets, electric fires, cookers and fridge freezers. While you cannot avoid having these items around you, you can be more aware of their effects and take some simple precautions to make your environment safer: keeping rooms well ventilated, not sitting too near the television set, taking frequent breaks from your VDU set and fitting a screen protector (see 'Useful Addresses').

Electrical pollution can be harmful to the body both because of the production of positive ions and also by the effect on the bio-electrical system.

Many people get headaches when there are changes in barometric pressure during hot, windy weather or during the full phase of the moon. Part of the problem is a high concentration of positive ions in the air. More about this follows.

## Ions

At the end of last century scientists discovered that air electricity comes from molecules or ions of gas; each molecule has a positively charged core of protons and neutrons surrounded by negatively charged electrons. In stable air there should be equal amounts so that they cancel each other out. In electrically unbalanced air, the electron, which is lighter, is displaced and an ion is created. So unbalanced air is made of molecules that have either lost or attracted a negative electron. If a molecule loses an electron it becomes positively charged. If the displaced electron attaches to a normal molecule, that molecule becomes negatively charged. The energy that disturbs normal air and creates charged molecules is radiation. In nature tiny amounts of radioactive substances come from the earth and the rays of the sun. Nature balances air at about five positive to four negative ions; 1000–2000 ions per cubic centimetre of air are necessary for healthy life. Scientific tests have proved that at levels significantly lower than this, plants and animals do not survive.[1]

Without ions we could not absorb oxygen in the quantities we need to function and it has been clearly demonstrated that the nervous system is calmer, sleeping is better and people are more cheerful where the concentration of negative ions is high.

## Disturbances of the Normal Electrical Charge of the Air

Hot winds, thundery conditions and electrical equipment can all overload the air with positive ions. When the moon is full, because a positively charged layer of air is pushed nearer to the earth, the number of positive ions increases. Air high in positive ions raises serotonin levels in the brain. Serotonin is an important neurohormone and its part in headaches and migraines has already been discussed. Overproduction of serotonin produces hyperactivity, followed by exhaustion, anxiety and depression. The increase in serotonin levels in weather-sensitive people can cause the 'serotonin irritation syndrome': migraine, hot flushes, irritability ('lunar madness'), sleeplessness, breathing problems, tension, anxiety, digestive problems, dry husky throats, itchy noses, swollen mucosa and conjunctivitis. Breathing air high in positive ions stimulates histamine production, which triggers allergies. This often leads people to believe the pollen count is high when in fact their problems are caused by air high in positive ions.

## Negative Ions

Negative ions reduce the amount of serotonin in the brain. Concentrations of negative ions are high in the country, particularly by running water, in mountainous areas, by the sea and even in the shower. Pollutants such as smoke destroy them immediately.

## Ionizers

These are machines which generate negative ions and clean the air. Domestic models are about the size of a small radio. There are smaller ones which fit into a car and much larger ones for industrial usage. Inside the plastic case a negative voltage is applied to sharp needles, causing a high-energy reaction to occur at the tip so that electrons are shot off at high velocity and collide with air molecules to form negative ions. These emerge from the ionizer in a stream. This stream, the 'ion wind', can be felt against the skin as a slight cool breeze. They are available in the electrical department of most good department stores or by mail order from health magazines. When positioning your ionizer make sure the air can circulate freely around it. Keep it away from the wall because the dust it extracts can cause discoloration; you might want to place a sheet of paper or cloth behind the ionizer on the stand to collect falling dust. Do not worry about this dust – it is better on the table than in your lungs.

# Daylight – Essential for Health

When looking at ways to improve the general health, the effect of daylight on the body is greatly underestimated. This is not only because changes in lifestyle have deprived a large proportion of the population of exposure to daylight but also because many people who are keen to get fit spend their time in indoor leisure complexes, weightlifting, doing aerobics and so on.

In the last decade, the effect of light on human health has been the subject of increasing scientific inquiry. Biologists have discovered that not only is it vital for our well-being, but also that individual requirements for light vary as much as individual needs for vitamins. As man has become more civilized he has spent less time outdoors, and many people travel to work by car to badly lighted buildings and then return home by car to spend an evening indoors watching television. Light deprivation in humans is not as obvious as in plants, which would wilt if placed in a dark corner, or as in some animals, which are full of energy at dawn and sleep at twilight, but there is no doubt that spending too much time indoors – and also the reduced light of the shorter days of autumn and winter – do adversely affect some people.

## How Does Light Affect the Body?

Daylight is necessary for normal brain functioning and for the regulation of the sleep–wake cycle. When daylight enters the eye it stimulates the pineal gland and inhibits the production of a substance called melatonin;* normally this is only produced at night in the dark. This is what makes us sleep. It also aids digestion and helps the production of vitamin D, and this, in turn, aids the absorption of calcium, phosphorus and magnesium.

## What Happens When We are Starved of Light

There is loss of concentration, the immune system becomes depleted and we feel lethargic, anxious and depressed. An extreme form of this is what is known as 'winter blues' or seasonal affective disorder (SAD). When the days shorten in autumn, sufferers experience symptoms which grow worse during winter, and they can be profoundly depressed. They also experience lethargy, loss of interest in sex, have joint pains and digestive problems, crave sweet foods and lack concentration to such a degree that they cannot continue their work or studies. They have great

* For information on melatonin supplementation contact New Nutrition (see Useful Addresses).

difficulty getting out of bed in the mornings and are exhausted all day. Their lack of concentration may be so severe that they have to abandon their studies or give up work. As spring approaches the symptoms abate and usually by May sufferers feel well, but are often very frustrated by the disruption in their lives and by the knowledge that they will have the same to face the following winter.

Fortunately, it has been found that being exposed, for several hours daily, to light which replicates daylight (full-spectrum light), cures this condition. This approach is now being used in hospitals in preference to drug-based therapy; even better news is that these lights are now available for large areas such as offices or therapy areas and also as small transportable units which can stand on a table for use in the home.

## Benefits in the Office – Reduction in Absenteeism and Improved Productivity

- Boosting of immune system reduces incidence of colds and flu.
- Helps to avoid onset of heart disease by dilating arteries and strengthening heart action.
- Helps depression by stimulating endocrine system and circulation.
- Helps fatigue by improving glucose metabolism and increasing blood flow to brain and muscles.
- Increased blood flow to brain helps concentration.
- Provides clearer illumination with high levels of definition and therefore reduces eye strain.

## Benefits in the Therapy Room

Simultaneous benefit to patient and therapist: when a unit was fitted in the Spar Clinic at Tring, workers were better able to maintain energy throughout the day and the incidence of coughs and colds decreased.

## Benefits in the Home

The unit can be used by the whole family. It is safe and no special goggles are needed. It is normally used for half an hour or one hour daily, but can also be used as background lighting. Weary housewives can relax in front of it when the children have gone to school, tired husbands can come home to it and students can do their homework in front of it.

The results with ME patients who use full-spectrum light daily are very encouraging.

To understand more about the importance of daylight see *Daylight Robbery: The Importance of Sunlight to Health* by Dr Damien Downing (Arrow, 1988).

For information on full-spectrum lighting:

Spectra Lighting Limited
York House
Harlestone
Northampton NN7 4EW
Tel: 01604 821904
Fax: 01604 821902.

## Sunlight

While it is foolish to risk skin cancer or ageing the skin prematurely from baking in the sun for hours, it is equally foolish never to allow the air and sun to reach the body. Frequent exposure for short periods has many beneficial effects, including the production of vitamin D. We look healthier after a little sun and this increases feelings of well-being. Sunlight also kills bacteria and fungus.

## The Sun Headache

This is a headache caused by the sun beating down on the top of the head; it is not caused by flickering sunlight, which can trigger migraine. You can avoid both types by wearing a hat and sunglasses.

## REFERENCES

1. Soyka, Fred, *The Ion Effect*, Bantam, 1978

## BIBLIOGRAPHY

Berger, B. G., and Owen, D. R., 'Mood alteration with swimming', *Psychosomatic Medicine*, 45 (1983), 425–33

Morgan, W. P., 'Anxiety reduction following acute physical activity', *Psychiatry Ann.*, 9 (1979), 141–7

Kripke, D. F., 'Therapeutic effects of light in depressed patients', *Ann. N Y Academy Science*, 435 (1985)

# 14

# The Electrical System of the Body

Some readers will want to dismiss this chapter as esoteric nonsense. That is unfortunate, for it is my belief that we cannot begin to comprehend and care for our total being without some openness to what cannot be seen, what is not in the pages of Gray's *Anatomy* or other tomes on classical medicine.

## Is Our Skin Really the Outer Limit of Our Being?

Mystics all over the world for five thousand years have believed that several layers of energy connect with the physical body and go beyond it, usually to an area of several feet or more. These layers have been called the etheric or subtle bodies.

Every living organism is surrounded by an energy field and we are no exception. Our brains, hearts, nerves and muscles all run on a subtle form of electricity which is discharged into the area surrounding the body; scientists call it the human energy field – others might call it the aura.

In the 1930s a Russian called Kirlian experimented with photography which clearly showed this field. One of the first people to study what he called the L-fields or the fields of life and how they affect health, was Harold Saxon Burr, of Yale University Medical School. Dr Robert O. Becker, author of *The Body Electric*, a leading modern researcher on electromagnetic pollution,

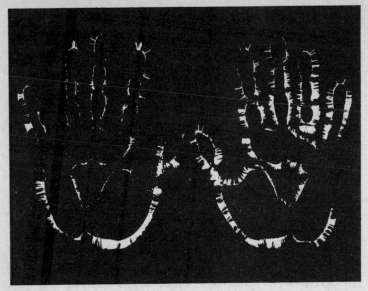

9. The energy field before and after a foot massage

believes that man-made electromagnetic fields from power lines and electrical appliances can affect the body and its surrounding energy field, and can cause physical and psychological problems. His research, and the research of others, suggests that disturbances in the electrical field develop before illness in the physical body. This could be the medicine of the future, the prevention and treatment of illness through correcting faults in the electromagnetic field.

## Therapeutic Touch

Dolores Kreiger, an American nurse, has worked very hard for twenty years teaching health professionals and lay people to use their hands to 'unruffle' the human energy field in order to bring comfort and healing to those in distress, whether it be to relieve a headache, to allow an anxious person to relax, to relieve the pain of muscle spasm, calm a crying baby or bring peace to the terminally ill and their relatives. She has called the technique, which was the subject of her doctorate, 'therapeutic touch'. This is somewhat of a misnomer because the person in distress is not actually touched: the helper's hands merely move in the energy field over the body surface at a distance of three to four inches from the body. She describes her simple technique in her book *The Therapeutic Touch — How to Use Your Hands to Help or Heal* (Prentice-Hall Inc.). One of her students, Janet Macrae, has written a perhaps more accessible book called *Therapeutic Touch* (Penguin). Medical personnel who have access to MEDLINE (Therapeutic Touch) will find a wealth of scientific references on this subject.

My advice is to read the book to get an idea of the technique, but *not* to expect to feel blocked, congested or depleted energy, or any energy described in any particular way. How your hands feel energy is *your* experience. You will develop your own system. Just follow the rules of relaxing, 'centring', trusting and working from the heart — the 'effortless effort'. Also remember that people who feel *nothing at all* in their hands can still be very effective in helping others.

## The Human Energy System and Health

While Western medicine concerns itself only with the functioning of the circulatory system, digestive system and so on, Eastern medicine (the principles of which are in many alternative therapies) also treats imbalances in the flow of energy in the body's meridians and in the energy field surrounding the body.

## The Meridians

These are the lines which allow ch'i (prana, universal energy) to flow around the body. There are twelve meridians particularly

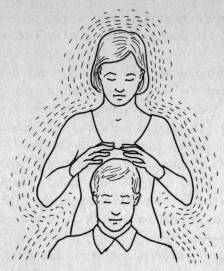

10. Working on the human energy field

associated with twelve organs or systems which run symmetrically on either side of the body. There are also two 'vessel' meridians running up the middle of the body – one on the front and one on the back.

## The Chakras

Chakra is a Sanskrit word meaning 'wheel'. The chakras of the body are similar to wheels in that they are spinning vortexes of energy. The human body contains hundreds of locations of concentrated energy but the main ones are in the midline of the body and extend from the crown to the base of the spine. They correspond to the major nerve plexuses of the physical body and each major chakra has its counterpart on the back of the body. There are several minor chakras, the most important of which are the feet chakras, through which we 'ground', and the hand chakras, which can be used to help or heal ourselves and others.

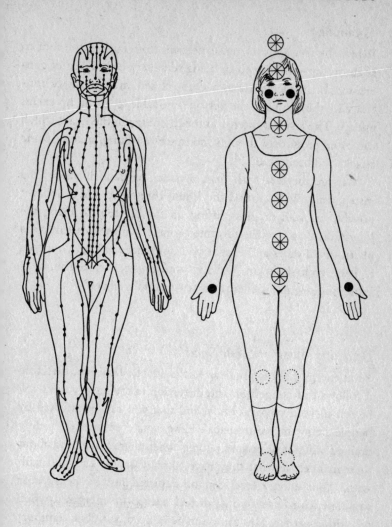

seven major chakras

subsidiary chakras

subsidiary chakras from behind

11. The acupuncture meridians  12. The location of the chakras

## Grounding

When the feet are very tense, perhaps from curling the foot to keep on slip-on shoes, from being sedentary or because of general tension, the feet chakras become closed through lack of contact with the earth and the person is not able to 'earth' his excess energy. The result is often too much energy in the head, which can cause pressure of thought, compulsive talking, anxiety, panic attacks and headaches.

Massage the feet with firm pressure, particularly under the instep, daily. Walk around the house barefooted and whenever possible on sand or grass, lifting up the big toes to bring the longitudinal arch of the foot into contact with the earth. Avoid plastic-soled shoes and ensure you don't need to curl your toes to keep your shoes on. Walking with the feet relaxed in well-fitting shoes is an excellent way to 'ground' yourself.

## Becoming Aware of 'Your Space'

Your energy field is physical – it is attached to you, therefore it follows that congestion and distortion in the energy field will be felt in your physical body, and that you can be affected by people being in 'your space'. Have you ever noticed feeling drained when near certain people, when there is nothing about their manner or what they have to say that you can find fault with? Your energy level can be depleted just by being near someone. Conversely you can feel relaxed or energized when near other people. This can often be noticed on public transport when not a word is spoken. Sitting next to some people you can feel perfectly comfortable and allow your body to relax next to theirs, while with another fellow traveller you can feel restless and uneasy and want to pull away into your own 'space'.

# Can I Feel My Own Energy Field?

It is always a great pleasure to do the following exercise with a group and see faces light up as they feel the energy increasing between their hands. If this is not your experience and you feel nothing or very little, do not be discouraged. It will come with practice. Only 1 per cent of people feel nothing at all. Some people feel tingling, warmth, a feeling of pulling in their palms or a sensation of resistance as though their hands are trying to squash a piece of firm foam rubber. First you need to centre yourself.

## Centring

Thought is energy and energy follows thought, so it is essential to use your head as well as your hands. Centring simply means consciously clearing your mind of the clutter of the day and finding your peaceful 'centre'.

1. Sit in an upright chair with your back straight but not tense, drop your shoulders and take a couple of slow breaths.

2. Visualize something that will 'anchor' you. It could be imagining a cord, rope or whatever going from just below your navel to the centre of the earth, or that you are wearing very heavy boots, or that you are a sturdy tree with roots growing deep into the earth: you can use any imagery which suggests that you are safe and centred.

3. When you are centred (don't worry if this does not happen immediately – just relax and it will come) *think* 'I am open to receive energy' and imagine you are breathing in bright white light.

## Building Up the Energy Field between Your Hands

1. Stretch your fingers out wide and become aware of the palm chakras.

2. Rub your hands together briskly for about fifteen seconds.

3. Hold the hands about 8 in (20 cm) apart and gradually bring them towards each other until they are about 1 in (3 cm) apart, but do not let them touch. The movement is that of slowly playing a concertina.

4. Separate the hands again, this time to about 6 m (15 cm) apart and then bring them towards each other, again without touching.

5. This time bring them together again and bounce them together; remember to keep the hands relaxed. You will feel a resistance, a feeling of pressure, between your hands.

6. Accept what you feel in your hands. If you wish, using your forefinger make a circle in the air about 1 in (3 cm) from your palm. Do you feel the circle tickle?

## When Your Hands are Energized

You can then use your hands to smooth your own field and remove excess positive ions, or you can use this energy to help someone else. When helping another person there must always be the *conscious* thought 'I wish to help.' If you work from the heart and add love for the person, even if they are a stranger, then the results can be very dramatic.

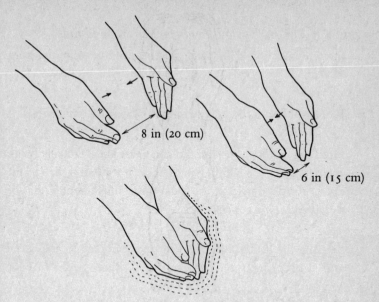

13. Building up the energy field between the hands

## *When You Feel a Headache Starting*

With your hands prepared as above:

1. Massage your feet (if possible with two or three drops of essential oil of lavender), paying particular attention to the part under the arch, for about 5 minutes for each foot.

2. Sit relaxed or lie on the floor or bed; slow down your breathing. With each out-breath imagine energy is leaving your head and travelling through the soles of your feet.

3. Reach up beyond your head and stroke about 3–4 in (8–10 cm) above your body just as though you were touching it –

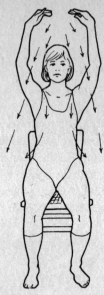

14. Clearing the energy field

down over your face, neck, chest and abdomen, and then sweep the hands to either side of the body; this is important because you need to take the congestion clear of your body. You will feel prickling or heat in your hands as you pick up congestion. You can just flick this off as though you were shaking water from your hands.

4. Continue stroking for about 10 minutes or until your arms feel tired. If you feel too unwell to make these movements just rest your hands on your head or hold them about 3 in (8 cm) away from your scalp.

5. Imagine your body and the area around your body to a distance of about 5 ft (1.5 m) is filled with white light.

## FURTHER READING

Brennan, Barbara Ann, *Hands of Light: A Guide to Healing through the Human Energy Field*, Bantam (New Age Books), 1988
This is a marvellous book, but it might be a little daunting for the beginner. Barbara Brennan has an impressive background. She was a research scientist for NASA at the Goddard Space Flight Center following completion of her MSc in atmospheric physics at the University of Wisconsin. For the past fifteen years she has been studying and working with the human energy field.

Bingham, W. E., Jr, 'Electromagnetic and electrostatic field: a neglected area in physiological psychology', *Journal of Psychology*, (1954), 225–31

Keller, Elizabeth, and Bzdek, Virginia M., 'Effect of therapeutic touch on tension headache pain', *Nursing Research*, 35, 2 (March/April 1986)

# PART THREE

# Alternative Therapies

There is often debate as to whether treatments other than allopathic medicine should be termed 'alternative' or 'complementary'. It would seem that there is a place for both terms, since some treatments are an adjunct to medical help and others are able to help or cure problems which medical science is unable to treat.

Space does not permit the inclusion of all the complementary or alternative treatments for headaches, such as biofeedback, herbal medicine (feverfew), Bach flower remedies, acupuncture, osteopathy, cranial osteopathy, the McTimmony Corley method of chiropractic, remedial massage, naturopathy and spiritual healing. You may want to explore one or more of these for yourself. Chapters on homoeopathy, shiatsu, reflexology and the Alexander Technique follow.

# 15

# Homoeopathy

Homoeopathic practitioners are often consulted by patients who suffer from chronic headaches or migraines. During the initial consultation, you will be asked about stress levels, dietary factors and your emotional well-being, and a detailed medical history will be taken. By gathering this information, the homoeopath attempts to gain a sense of the patient as an individual, with a view to selecting the appropriate homoeopathic medicine. Most practitioners will also make additional suggestions regarding positive changes in personal habits that will support homoeopathic treatment. This may involve exploring relaxation techniques, learning positive ways of managing stress, or making obvious dietary adjustments.

## Selecting a Homoeopathic Remedy

For a homoeopathic remedy to be effective, it must fit the precise symptoms of each individual patient as accurately as possible. The remedy acts as a catalyst, giving the body the boost that is needed for the symptoms to be resolved.

In the case of a headache, it is necessary to obtain detailed information about the nature of the pain (shooting, throbbing, bursting, etc.), where it is located (side of the head, above the eyes, back of the head, etc.), what makes it better or worse, and if any other symptoms have set in before or since the headache began (nausea, dizziness, irritability, light sensitivity, flushed or pale skin, etc.). Once this information is obtained, it is possible to decide which homoeopathic remedy fits the symptoms as a whole most closely.

Above all, it is essential to remember that the relevant symptoms are those that have arisen since the illness began. In other words, if someone is normally pale, this would not be listed as a symptom. However, if the patient normally has a rosy complexion and has become very pale and drawn since pain set in, this becomes a relevant factor when choosing the appropriate homoeopathic remedy.

## What to Expect: Possible Reactions to a Homoeopathic Remedy

If the selected homoeopathic medicine bears little resemblance to the symptoms of the patient, there will be no improvement. On the other hand, if the remedy is very close, but not a perfect match, there is likely to be marginal improvement. Once an accurate match has been established between the symptoms of the patient and the appropriate remedy, the result should be a decisive and rapid improvement of symptoms, as well as a general feeling of enhanced well-being.

## Deciding When Home Prescribing is Appropriate

Assessing when to consult a homoeopath for treatment and when to try self-help prescribing is reasonably simple. In general, conditions that are categorized as *acute* are appropriate for self-help. Problems that fall into this category are short-lived, self-limiting (have a predictable time span) and tend to clear up of their own accord given appropriate conditions for recovery. Good examples include colds, influenza, coughs, food poisoning, cuts and bruises.

Problems that are not suitable for home prescribing are those that are classed as *chronic* conditions. These are long-term health problems that do not resolve themselves, but are subject to regular flare-ups of the condition. They include arthritis, eczema, asthma, hay fever, stomach ulcers, migraines and sinusitis. These conditions require skilled case management for the most positive outcome. As a result, they are best treated by a homoeopathic practitioner who is likely to have the necessary skill and experience to decipher what is happening in a complicated case at any given time.

If we take on board the information given above regarding acute and chronic conditions, it becomes clear that migraines and recurrent headaches are best treated by a homoeopathic practitioner. However, if an isolated headache occurs as a result of overindulgence in alcohol, an unusually stressful event or lack of sleep, it may be classed as an acute episode which may be appropriately dealt with by home prescribing.

## How to Obtain Homoeopathic Remedies

Homoeopathic medicines can be easily purchased from homoeopathic pharmacies, health food stores and high-street chemists. The potency (strength) of medicines that is most readily available over the counter is the sixth centesimal potency (usually labelled 6c). This is a perfectly appropriate strength for the beginner to use. As experience is gained in homoeopathic prescribing stronger potencies may be obtained from homoeopathic pharmacies. However, it is suggested that the home prescriber should not go above a 12c or 30c potency, since these should be adequate for straightforward acute conditions. Homoeopathic remedies are most commonly obtained in tablet form, but they can also be taken in the form of powders, granules or capsules, or in liquid suspension. Creams, ointments, tinctures and lotions for external use only may also be purchased.

## *How to Take Homoeopathic Medicines*

Once the appropriate remedy has been selected, take two tablets (this is the first dose). The tablets should be chewed or sucked rather than being washed down with water, since they need to be absorbed through the membranes of the mouth.

Since it is important to avoid contaminating the tablets by over-handling them, tip them on to a clean teaspoon before taking them. Also ensure that there are no strong flavours in the mouth that might interfere with the action of the remedy. The best way of ensuring this is to take homoeopathic medicine half an hour before or after eating or drinking.

Some substances are thought to interfere with the curative potential of homoeopathic remedies. These include tea, coffee, peppermint, camphor and eucalyptus, and aromatic inhalations such as Olbas Oil.

After taking the first dose, wait for an hour before assessing any response. If there has been a marked improvement, do not repeat the remedy unless and until symptoms return. On the other hand, if a slight, short-lived change for the better has occurred, take a second dose of the selected remedy. When no improvement occurs, or the symptoms have changed, check whether another remedy may now be more appropriate.

Always remember that homoeopathic medicines should be taken on a short-term basis only. Once an improvement has set in, it is very important to stop taking the medication. This is done in order to allow the body to rectify the situation by itself. If it becomes necessary to take regular doses of a homoeopathic remedy in order to sustain an improvement, this is an indication that self-help measures are not appropriate and that professional homoeopathic advice is needed in order to address the under-lying disorder that is leading to the problem.

Most important of all, if there is any doubt or confusion or anxiety about home prescribing, always seek a professional opinion rather than soldiering on alone.

## Commonly Indicated Homoeopathic Remedies for Headaches

The following list includes some of the most frequently used homoeopathic medicines for headaches. The remedy which fits the symptoms most accurately will provide the greatest relief. However, if headaches are a recurrent problem, it is best to seek professional advice.

### Belladonna

Headaches that respond best to belladonna are characteristically of sudden, violent onset and may follow overexposure to sunlight or chill. Pains are usually right-sided and of a throbbing, pulsating nature. There is general sensitivity to light, noise and movement, which make pains and discomfort worse. Relief is obtained from lying propped up in a quiet, darkened room or bending the head backwards.

### Bryonia

Headaches arise as a result of a generally unwell state, often linked to constipation. Symptoms develop slowly and insidiously with pains affecting the forehead or nape of the neck. A nauseating dizziness may accompany the headache, which is made worse by the slightest movement. Warmth also makes the pain worse, while keeping still, cool air and firm pressure improve the situation.

### Nux vomica

Indicated for 'morning-after' headaches, which are brought on by overindulgence in alcohol and food; also for stress-induced, tension headaches with reliance on coffee, alcohol or painkillers to keep going. Pains are worst on waking, getting better as the day goes on. Constipation and nausea accompany the headache, which is made worse by stress, mental effort, lack of sleep, noise and anger. Warmth, peace and quiet, resting and sound sleep are soothing.

## Lachesis

Treats left-sided headaches that come on after sleep. Bursting pains extend from the left eye to the nose. Dizziness with headache is made worse by closing the eyes and looking steadily at one object. Feels generally worse from tight or restrictive clothing around the waist. Pains are aggravated by sleep, heat, sunlight, alcohol, movement and closing eyes; they are relieved by fresh air, cool compresses and pressure.

## Gelsemium

Appropriate for dizzy, sick headache with band-like pressure around the forehead. Tense feeling may also extend from the crown of the head to the shoulder. Congested sensation in the head, with very sensitive scalp. Headaches may be brought on by anticipating an important event. Pains are made worse by stress, movement, humidity, smoking, hot, sunny weather and thundery conditions. They are relieved by sweating, bending forwards, resting with the head supported and passing copious amounts of urine.

# Homoeopathic Remedies for Migraines

Any of the following remedies, or those listed above, may be of help in an acute episode of migraine, provided the symptoms match those of the patient. However, if migraines are severe, well-established or happen at regular intervals, treatment should be obtained from a homoeopathic practitioner.

## Sanguinaria

Indicated for right-sided migraines with pains that radiate from the base of the skull over the right eye. Headache occurs from low blood sugar levels as a result of skipping meals. Pulsating pains increase at night, and are made worse from jarring movements, too much sugar and bright light. They are relieved by sleep, cool air and vomiting.

## Iris

Blurred vision precedes migraine; nauseating headache with tiredness and shooting pains in temples; scalp feels tight and contracted. Pains are worse from coughing, exposure to cool air and mental exhaustion, and they are relieved by gentle movement.

## Nat. mur. (Natrum muriaticum)

Taken for migraine with visual disturbance and numbness or tingling of the face and lips. Bursting pains settle over the eyes, or on the crown of the head. Headache is worse on waking, exposure to bright sunlight, before or after a period, reading or movement of any kind. The pain is relieved by fresh air, cool bathing, resting and keeping as still as possible.

## Sepia

For migraines with shooting pains that lodge over the left eye. Unpleasant heavy sensations in the crown of the head with dizziness, nausea and possibly vomiting. Feeling washed out and exhausted. Symptoms seem worse for sitting still indoors, and better for exercise in the fresh air. Stooping, kneeling, jarring movements and the premenstrual period all make symptoms worse. Warmth, sleep and open air result in general improvement.

Thank you to Beth MacEoin for her chapter on homoeopathy. Beth is a practising homoeopath/writer and lives in the north-east of England.

## USEFUL ADDRESSES

A list of professional homoeopaths may be obtained from:
The Society of Homoeopaths
2 Artizan Road
Northampton NN1 4HU
Tel: 01604 21400

A list of orthodox doctors who have obtained a postgraduate qualification in homoeopathy may be obtained from:
The British Homoeopathic Association
27a Devonshire Street
London WC1N 3HZ
Tel: 0171 935 2163

Homoeopathic remedies are available in many pharmacies.

## FURTHER READING

Castro, Miranda, *The Complete Homoeopathy Handbook: A Guide to Everyday Healthcare*, Macmillan, 1990

Cunnings, Stephen, and Ullman, Dana, *Everybody's Guide to Homoeopathic Medicines: Taking Care of Your Family with Safe and Effective Remedies*, Gollancz, 1986

MacEoin, Beth, *Homoeopathy*, Hodder & Stoughton, 1992

Ullman, Dana, *Homoeopathy, Medicine for the Twenty-first Century*, Thorsons, 1985

# 16

# *Shiatsu*

Shiatsu is a form of oriental massage. Literally translated from Japanese, it means 'finger pressure', although in practice we use varying degrees of pressure from the fingers, thumbs, palms of the hands, elbows or even the feet. In addition, the more mobile techniques such as kneading, stretching or rotating are used.

Shiatsu is based on an understanding of the human body as a dynamic system of energy which circulates in channels called meridians, activating and charging the body organs and their functions. With shiatsu, the flow of this energy is stimulated and harmonized to create a balancing of these functions and awaken the body's natural healing process. Pressure on specific points not only releases hormones, including natural painkillers, but improves the circulation of blood and lymph and affects the nervous system.

## Intuitive 'Shiatsu'

You may have squeezed the bridge of your nose or massaged your temples attempting to relieve a headache. If you have an ache or pain perhaps you have felt around for some pressure point that will induce a 'good hurt', the pain that makes the pain go away. If you bump into something you may instinctively put your hand to that injured part, giving firm, squeezing, supportive pressure to neutralize the pain. It is as if, by focusing attention in that area, self-healing is activated.

All of these intuitive responses work like shiatsu. They are all ways of adjusting our own energy system, of changing how we are inside from our outside.

## Daily Energy Adjustments

Every day we are constantly adjusting our energy by what we eat and drink, by activities like walking, running, talking, resting, reading, driving, singing, laughing, shouting and so on, by the way in which we breathe, the company we keep or the climate we experience. These adjustments affect our energy in an endless variety of ways, to energize or relax us, to settle or unsettle us, to make us more outwardly or inwardly orientated, etc.

Such constant adaptations form the rhythm of our lives. They are our conscious and unconscious means of creating balance within ourselves, and are our primary healthcare. Following nature's cycles we work, and then rest and play and are renewed. We then work again. However, sometimes following work comes more work, or arguing or worry; or mental activity is not followed by physical action but by more heady situations. We do the same to our bodies: for example, when our system needs to be alkaline we may not understand and eat more acid-forming foods instead. When we live like this, we become one-sided and then symptoms of imbalance are inevitable. For example, if you work outdoors in the cold in circumstances of responsibility, are constrained by time, feel under pressure and your diet is high in animal food and salt, then the balance of your energy is downward – to contract, make tight and harden. This can cause tension in the neck and give rise to dull, heavy headaches at the back of your head. It may be possible to find relief by resting somewhere warm and comfortable. Alternatively, if you work in a warm, stuffy environment your activities are more mentally and emotionally oriented. Add to this lots of tea or coffee and refined or sugary foods and this emphasizes more upward-moving, expanding energy. The result can be times when you cannot stop thinking and other times when you cannot think. Sometimes you may feel your head is going to burst and you experience a throbbing or explosive pain to the front of your head. Even simply taking a gentle walk in the fresh air can help to restore balance.

## Using Shiatsu

Shiatsu is a powerful way to access our energy system and effect change within us. Some techniques can be practised on yourself, but for others you will need the help of a friend or a shiatsu practitioner. Since there are many types of headaches with numerous origins you will have to experiment to find which points and methods are most effective. Try a few *tsubos* (pressure points), searching for those which you feel connect with your pain. Use your thumb, index or middle finger, pressing with the area between the tip and the pad. Just how hard to press and for how long will be different in each instance. Apply the pressure slowly until you reach that point somewhere between pain and pleasure: a 'good hurt'. If you sustain this then the pain should begin to fade away.

### Use the Following Points for Headache

Large intestine #4, on the back of each hand in the centre of the fleshy part between the thumb and index finger, pushing towards the bone of the index finger.

Large intestine #11; when you bend your elbow at 90° there is a crease on the front of your arm.

The point directly between the eyebrows called *In Do*, and also on the temples, either by pressure or circular massage using two fingers.

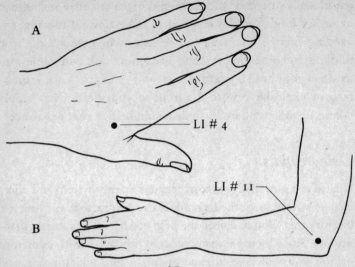

15. Shiatsu pressure points, A and B

On the back of the neck, Governing Vessel #15 on the mid-line between the base of the skull and the hairline (the space between the first and second cervical vertebrae). Also, just below the skull, 1 in (3 cm) either side of the midline, the points Bladder #10, and at 2 in (5 cm) either side, Gall Bladder #20.

## For Sinus Blockage and Facial Tension

Large intestine #20 on the face in the small grooves to the outside of each nostril (figure C). Also to ease facial tension you can use Stomach #3 directly below the centre of each eye just under the cheek-bone. An alternative technique is to give deep pulsing pressure. For pain to one side of the front of the head, on that same side work on Large Intestine #4 (figure A), pressing in and slightly towards the arm and on the head; also Gall Bladder #14 (figure C) 1 in (3 cm) above the centre of the eyebrow, pushing inwards and upwards.

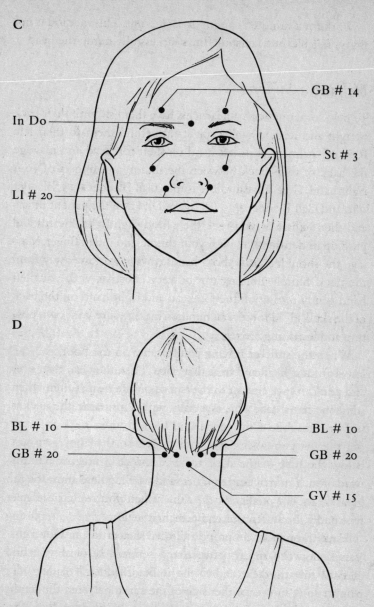

C

GB # 14

In Do

St # 3

LI # 20

D

BL # 10

BL # 10

GB # 20

GB # 20

GV # 15

16. Shiatsu pressure points, C and D

Work for a minute at a time at each point. This method is not always reliable, but can sometimes successfully numb the head.

## Helping a Sufferer

To help someone with a headache, have them sit with their back straight and relaxed while you stand behind them to their left. Rest the palm of your left hand on their forehead and massage the back of their neck between the thumb and fingers of your right hand. Give shiatsu to the tsubos Gall Bladder #15, Bladder #10 and Gall Bladder #20 (all figure D). Have the patient inhale and then exhale as you rock their head slightly backwards and push up under the skull with your thumb and index finger. Massage the shoulders using both hands, always working away from the neck. Simply holding can be very effective, with your left hand gently resting on the forehead and right hand on the back of the skull. Hold for several minutes, making sure your own posture and breathing are relaxed.

When the sufferer is lying comfortably on the floor, you can kneel at their head and treat their face. Then they can turn over and you can give shiatsu to the tsubos on the head. Often when someone has a headache, especially with a migraine, the neck is stiff or immobile. Cup your hands beneath their neck and ease out the neck muscles. Curl your fingers so that they grip just below the base of the skull and pull the skull horizontally towards you. You may find tightness and swelling here and a rough, greasy, rubbery quality to the skin. When you stretch the area repeatedly the sufferer often finds great relief.

Have the patient lie prone and give shiatsu to the Governor Vessel #14, the space between the seventh cervical vertebra and the first thoracic; and to the tsubos Bladder #19 (for side pain), 1 in (3 cm) on either side of the space between the tenth and eleventh thoracic vertebrae and also to Bladder #21 (for

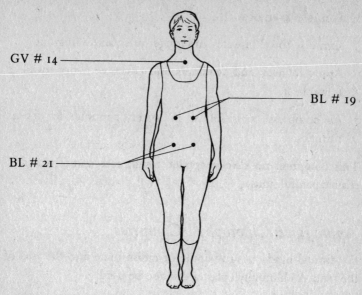

GV # 14

BL # 19

BL # 21

17. Shiatsu pressure points

frontal pain). These are positioned 1 in (3 cm) either side of the space between the twelfth thoracic and the first lumbar vertebrae.

## Ginger Compress

In addition to using our hands, there are other external applications which can be most effective. Here is the method for making a ginger compress:

1. Grate a piece of root ginger 2–3 in (5–8 cm) long.

2. Wrap in a muslin or thin cotton sock.

3. Place in a large pan of water and slowly heat this to just before boiling point.

4. Remove from heat.

5. Immerse towel in water and ginger juice and wring out.

6. Apply to neck and shoulders and cover with dry towel to retain heat.

7. As compress cools reheat in water; continue for 15–20 minutes.

This compress can also be applied to the face and forehead to relieve painful sinuses.

## Apple Juice; Chlorophyll Compress

For frontal headaches rub apple or radish juice into the area of the pain. A chlorophyll plaster can also be used:

1. Chop and crush cabbage and mix to a paste with a little white flour.

2. Spread mixture ½ in (1 cm) thick on a paper towel and apply to the head with the mixture next to the skin for an hour or two.

Headaches deep inside or towards the back of the head may improve if you drink warm apple juice. Sharper-tasting apples are more effective.

## Diet and Lifestyle

As mentioned before, you will have to experiment to gain a dynamic grasp of how to access and adjust your condition. The first step is to look at how you are influencing your energies by the foods you are giving your body to work on.

With *frontal headaches* avoid sugar, coffee, fruit juice, processed foods, alcohol and excessive liquid. *Sinus* sufferers should avoid mucus-forming foods such as flour and dairy products. With headaches at the *side of the head* be wary of fats and oils, and with headaches *deep inside the head* avoid eggs, red meat and salty foods.

When trying to resolve your headaches don't just look as far as the symptoms. Try instead to see what the symptom is showing you about the overall direction of your energy, and use this to guide you towards a more balanced diet and lifestyle for your future.

*

This chapter is by Paul Lambeth who has been a macrobiotic shiatsu practitioner for sixteen years. He also teaches at the Kushi Institute and the Community Health Foundation in London.

## FOR MORE INFORMATION

Community Health Foundation
188 Old Street
London EC1U 9BP
Tel: 0171 251 4076

The Shiatsu Society
19 Langside Park
Kilbarchan
Renfrewshire PA10 2EP

# 17

# Reflexology

Reflexology emerges from an ancient philosophy that grasps a fundamental awareness of the essence of being – a whole can only be separated with some dis-ease; for equilibrium and balance the whole body has to be recognized for what it truly is, a vehicle for physical, emotional, mental and spiritual expression. Holistic therapies, such as reflexology, base all their teaching on the acceptance of energy flow. For a physical entity to sustain life it must have energy; the three components of the atoms of which we are all made are held together and supported by energy. Disease and poor vitality are merely signals that the body uses to communicate to us that some element of our being is not balanced, is not synchronized. The body is only as strong as its weakest organ and a block on one level will inevitably create a block on another. We then develop signs and symptoms and create a complicated picture that we then call ill health. Reflexology is a 'tool' that can be instrumental in correcting these imbalances simply by recognizing the connection between energy flow and well-being. A circulation free of blockage maintains health and vitality.

Reflexology aims to trigger the return of homeostasis, a balance of the internal organs. The feet are a microcosm of the body; they reflect every organ and structure as well as reiterating the energy pathways, and they are particularly sensitive because of their abundance of nerve endings. It is these nerve endings that are stimulated in a reflexology treatment. Nerves conduct electrochemical impulses or messages; they are channels of energy that connect the feet to the rest of the body. Massaging reflexes on the foot elicits a response in the glands and organs. The nerve impulses initiated by pressing reflex areas on the feet activates the autonomic nervous system. In health this amazing network of mutual antagonists manages the effects of stress and in turn activates many more networks. However, too much stimulation or stress of the system will eventually lead to exhaustion. It is only in a relaxed state that brain activity is reduced and the oscillations slow down. For a short time life stops throwing stimuli and the autonomic nervous system stops responding; a quiet mind has an awareness of its 'being' rather than its 'doing'. The major aim of any reflexology treatment is to induce relaxation – the physiological and psychological effects cannot be separated. To knit the two together brings the rewards of improved health and vitality.

## Headaches

The cause of a migraine headache at the site within the brain is thought to be a localized vasodilation causing an increase in pressure and consequently swelling. As the cranial nerves become affected problems are referred to eyes, ears, liver and stomach. Hypertension is also associated with headaches, as are dehydration caused by excess alcohol and stimulants, and hormonal and blood glucose imbalances. All these symptoms are interrelated, and a fine line between balance and imbalance may be triggered by any one of them. For example, glucose is almost the only fuel required by nerve tissue, and the body gives priority to the brain and the nervous system, so when blood glucose levels drop, the blood *volume* increases to compensate. If this mechanism is triggered too regularly, nerve tissue becomes over-sensitive to the pressure of the bulging blood vessels and so a headache is created.

Stress is probably most frequently blamed for headaches. It is estimated that 65 per cent of illness is stress-related. Stress can be defined as an internal response made to external changes and difficulties, whether real or imaginary. We experience stress when we lose faith in our ability to handle difficult situations. Recognized by the medical profession as the most effective treatment for stress is relaxation – a skilful exercise for the mind to find silence and stillness. A completely relaxed body cannot feel stress, cannot feel the negative emotions of anxiety, fear, pain or hatred; it may recognize the words but does not experience the emotion.

Reflexology massage encourages calm in the autonomic nervous system, and so its connecting networks are also calmed and its self-regulating mechanism is brought into balance.

One great advantage of reflexology is that painful or tender areas of the body need not be directly touched. Relief can be given by remote application.

## Using Reflexology

The numbers refer to the diagram on opposite page.

### Solar Plexus Reflex (1)

The solar plexus is a nerve network that supplies the abdominal organs. Situated behind the stomach and in front of the diaphragm, it is often referred to as the abdominal brain or 'nerve switchboard', for it relays fight-or-flight instructions from the brain to the adrenal glands. It aids movement of food through the stomach and small intestine, stimulates the liver in its

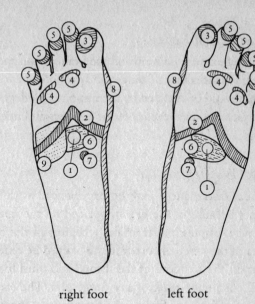

1. solar plexus
2. diaphragm
3. head/brain
4. eye/ear
5. sinus
6. pancreas
7. adrenals
8. spine
9. liver

right foot      left foot

18. Reflexology sites

bile-producing and detoxifying role, and sends messages to the kidneys to remove waste. This reflex is most useful for inducing a relaxed state. It can relieve stress and nervousness, aid deep breathing and restore calm.

## Diaphragm Reflex (2)

The diaphragm is the most important muscle for breathing, and is generally not used to its full capacity. Deep breathing (diaphragmatic breathing) should be encouraged to increase lung capacity and aid the exchange of oxygen and carbon dioxide from the cells. The connection between regular deep breathing and headaches is of the utmost importance (see section on aftercare below).

## Brain/Head Reflex (3)

The reflexes of the head and the brain are on the pads of the big toes. This area may be tender, and pressure and frequency of massage should be dictated by the response. Reflexes for the sides of the face are on the sides of the big toes and neck reflexes at the base.

## Eye/Ear Reflexes (4)

Visual disturbances may be experienced with migraine headaches because of the pressure placed on the optic nerve, which conveys impressions from the receptors in the eye to the visual area of the cerebral cortex in the brain. The reflexes are on both feet on the cushions of the second and third toes. Massage here will encourage relief of any congestion. The ear is not only the organ of hearing, for it also plays a part in maintaining balance, and disturbances here may be experienced with severe headaches. The reflexes are found on both feet on the cushions of the fourth and fifth toes.

## Sinus Reflexes (5)

The sinuses are cavities within the skull bones which communicate with the nasal cavities through small openings. They act as protection for the eyes and the brain and give resonance to the voice. Massage to the reflexes situated on the tip of the toes encourages the sinuses to flush out accumulated debris that builds up internal pressure.

## Pancreas Reflex (6)

A large glandular structure in the abdomen, the pancreas produces the hormones insulin and glucagon, which are important in the control of sugar metabolism.

## Adrenal Glands (7)

Situated at the upper tip of each kidney, the adrenal glands perform numerous vital functions related to physiological and psychological stress responses and are therefore important when dealing with headaches. They are divided into two parts: first, the cortex, which produces steroid hormones controlling the reabsorption of sodium and water in the kidneys as well as secreting potassium and sex hormones; secondly, the medulla, which produces adrenalin and noradrenalin, working in conjunction with the sympathetic nervous system. Adrenalin output is increased at times of anxiety and stress, and is responsible for the chain reaction in the fight-or-flight situation.

## Spinal Cord (8)

The curves of the inside of the foot correspond to the spine. The spine is the central support to the body and carries its weight. It is an important axis of movement. The spinal cord, enclosed by the bony structures of the column, carries the nerves from the brain to all parts of the body. Massage of this reflex sends signals to the surrounding muscles to relax. On this inside curve of the foot, attention is also given to the neck reflex at the base of the big toe, as well as the shoulder reflexes a little further along, to enable a free flow of energy to the head.

## Liver Reflex (9)

Finally, treatment of headaches cannot be discussed without giving attention to the liver reflex. The largest and most complex organ in the body, the liver takes a major role in detoxifying the blood and manufacturing bile for fat digestion.

## *Aftercare*

As mentioned, reflexology embraces a holistic philosophy and involves more than a foot massage. Any symptoms of imbalance require attention on all levels. The mental and emotional bodies are a continuum of the physical body and deserve recognition and support. Relaxation is all part of the reflexology treatment, but aftercare and maintenance are just as valuable. With practice, relaxation and deep breathing become automatic and should be incorporated in the management of headaches; they may be used as coping strategies. A quiet mind allows access to the sub-conscious and enables us to explore the roots of our emotions and behaviour. During deep relaxation or at lowered levels of consciousness, affirmation of positive thought may be seeded. We are what we think and feeding the subconscious with posit-ive energy eventually spills over into our conscious or awakened state and shows itself in our day-to-day existence. During relax-ation we release the 'struggle' and accept the free flow of energy physically, emotionally and mentally. This energy is our life force and the life force is our spirituality. The 'whole' has been addressed.

## *Deep Breathing and Relaxation Techniques*

One of the most important features of deep breathing is the fact that the respiratory muscles are fully called into play, and so not only ventilate and cleanse the lungs and the rest of the body, but also ventilate and cleanse the mind. Deep breathing refreshes the whole.

Man in his normal state has no need of instruction in breath-ing. However, he has constructed improper methods and atti-tudes of walking, standing and sitting, and in turn inhibited natural deep breathing. Consequently the flow of vital force has decreased. We therefore have to focus the mind until it remembers to do it by itself.

1.  Stand or sit erect. Breathing through the nostrils, inhale steadily, first filling the lower part of the lungs. This exerts a gentle pressure on the abdominal organs, pushing forward the front walls of the abdomen. Then fill the middle part of the lungs, pushing out the lower ribs, breastbone and chest. Now fill the higher portion of the lungs, lifting the chest. It may appear that the breathing consists of three distinct movements, but with practice becomes a steady continuous action. The one inhalation should only take a couple of seconds.

2.  Retain the breath for a few seconds.

3.  Exhale quite slowly. When the air is entirely exhaled relax the chest and abdomen.

Regular practice of deep breathing automatically induces a relaxed state: at this point visualization and affirmation of thought may be introduced.

1.  Concentrate on allowing pure white light to penetrate the point of discomfort. Allow the light to absorb the block and as it does this imagine energy being allowed to flow freely around the entire body.

2.  Place an affirmation within the mind to serve the body, for example: 'This day is mine. I am in control of my time. My energies are centred and balanced. Nothing in my environment now or at any time can change that. All is well.'

3.  Affirm that you are willing to release the need for disease and in return accept the need for physical, emotional, mental and spiritual well-being.

This chapter has been contributed by Andrea Warwick RCT-MCIA, M Phys, MIFA.

## FOR MORE INFORMATION

British Reflexology Association
Monks Orchard
Whitbourne
Worcester SR6 5RB

# 18

# *The Alexander Technique*

The Alexander Technique can help all those people whose headaches are brought on by the way they have learnt to react to the events in the world in which they live. This, however, doesn't limit our scope too much. Headache caused by organic disease is, fortunately, very rare, although when it occurs, it is likely to be very serious,[1] needing expert, and perhaps urgent, medical care. So if, for the present article, we leave out those headaches caused by disease, tumours, fever, poisoning by toxic substances and perhaps eye strain, we are still left with the vast majority of headaches! Please notice that I am not claiming that we Alexander teachers cure headaches. Because headaches happen to people – in fact to people who have learned to have headaches – what we do is to help those people, should they wish, to learn how not to have headaches. It is a commonplace that, if someone comes to an Alexander lesson with a headache, they are likely to leave without it and, more importantly, as lessons continue, become less and less prone to headache until the headaches vanish altogether.

Let me explain how the technique helps. If a car or other machine was out of adjustment, even slightly, its performance would be affected all the time it was being used. It is the same for us, but with a fundamental difference: we create our own lack of adjustment by the way we react to all the stimuli of the world. As is stressed elsewhere in this book, headaches happen to people. In fact, as I will explain later, they happen to people who are out of shape. Therefore, we need to answer three questions.

1. How does the situation of almost universal poor shape come about?

2. What are the effects of being out of shape and, in particular, what is the link with headaches?

3. What can we do to change it?

## 1. How Do We Get Out of Shape?

You may not be aware of it, but you are 'using' yourself as a whole at this moment while reading this book. It is a safe assumption on my part because we do everything as a whole and 'use' ourselves in everything that we do. Furthermore, you are likely to be working far too hard – using too much muscular effort – while you are reading, again without knowing it.

In exactly the same way that we have to learn to use tools, etc., we have to learn to use ourselves. This includes being upright and moving, as well as all of those activities in which we may think that our individuality can more easily be seen – speaking, writing, drawing, etc. In short, everything that we do is learned and involves brain activity, whether we are aware of it or not. Much of early learning is likely to involve imitating the people around us. We have already noted that most people seem to pull themselves out of shape – 'pull down' as F. M. Alexander called it – so we are likely to copy that. Alexander's description of pulling down is very vivid. It is as though we had a rope around our neck, the rope then passing through a massive ring screwed into the floor and the free end being held in our hands. As we exert ourselves and pull on the rope we pull our neck forward, at the same time as pulling our head backwards and down at the top of the neck. The lower back is unduly arched, which has the effect of throwing the chest diagonally up. The legs are very stiff, with the joints braced. Being upright should be much more of a balancing act than most people realize and actually requires very little effort.[2] If you work too hard just to stay upright, the more you exert yourself, the greater the pulling down. What is more, as we are not very good at 'letting go' after activity, it is as if the rope was shortened a little every day – the pulling down increases gradually. On top of this we overlay our own personal tensions: clenching the fists, curling the toes, frowning, pulling the tummy in, tightening the jaw and perhaps grinding the teeth. The list could go on. These represent our personal reactions to the stimuli of life, ranging from just staying upright to the most demanding of situations. The stimulus may be internal (from the 'mind' or from the 'body') or external, but either way, if you pull down, extra activity inevitably leads to more pulling down. It is a constant factor, affecting us in everything that we do, and generally totally hidden from us because it is present all the time. So the distortion of pulling down is caused by using more muscular effort than we need; indeed, we could call it misuse. Considering that we're all built on the same pattern, it's not really surprising that, fundamentally, we all seem to distort ourselves in much the same way.

## 2. What are the Effects of Being Out of Shape?

Working harder than we need – with the relativity of various parts of the body altered for the worse – makes us unnecessarily tired. However, particularly significant for headache is interference both with the blood supply to the brain and with breathing.

Firstly, pulling the head back and the neck forwards can put pressure on the carotid and vertebral arteries – the only blood-supply route to the brain.[3] If the blood flow to the brain is reduced to critical levels, all sorts of symptoms, common in headache sufferers, are experienced. As for breathing, when you pull yourself out of shape you will fix your ribs and interfere with what should be an automatic process of breathing in and out. This interference doesn't just happen when you are awake. If it takes place when you are asleep, especially deeply asleep, you may wake with a 'carbon dioxide' headache. This seems to be especially the case for people with cluster headaches.[4] Strange as it may seem, we are probably only free from pulling down while dreaming, when the muscles are almost totally relaxed.[5]

## 3. What Can be Done?

I have asserted that most headaches are caused by pulling down. The reason for my confidence is a practical one: pupils tend to become free from headaches in the course of lessons. The problem we have to solve is that of misuse on a habitual basis. In lessons, Alexander teachers have three main intentions: first, to get the pupil to be upright with the minimum of effort and teach the pupil how not to interfere with it; second, to teach the pupil how to make effort without pulling down; and third, to teach how it is possible to deal with the genuinely unpleasant stimuli of life without pulling down. This often requires a change of point of view on the part of the pupil. It is when we change our viewpoint and see that we must reject pulling down as being a necessary or desirable way of being in the world that we begin to have success. How easy this is and how long it takes depends on the individual, but forty half-hour lessons over a year will see most pupils on the right track. Twenty hours is, after all, less time than it takes most people to learn to drive.

You may have noticed that earlier, after excluding the sort of headaches that Alexander Technique can't help with, I did not then differentiate between other types such as migraine, tension headache, mixed headache and cluster headache. This was not in order to be vague or inaccurate, but rather born out of practicalities. Teaching the pupil how not to pull down is successful in combating headache no matter what the technical description. For us, it follows that the different types form a 'continuum'.

We are convinced that, whatever the specific mechanism of the pain of headaches, the initial factor is depriving the brain of blood by means of pulling down in reaction to life's events. While most people seem to pull down it is neither necessary nor good for us. Just being told, or even working out for ourselves, that we don't need to react in a particular way doesn't seem to make much difference. Why is that? Well, we must always remember that 'once makes a habit' and having established a way of reacting which includes pulling down – perhaps in such a way as to give ourselves a headache – that habit is always there. All that is necessary is for us to perceive the situation in our usual way.

Helping people to change the way they react is central to Alexander Technique, and so headaches which are a by-product of the way we live our life can disappear as a beneficial by-product of changing the way we react. It is in this way that Alexander Technique is therapeutic.

In summary, then, non-malign headache is self-created. It is not created out of stupidness, weakness of character or general worthlessness. Its source is pulling down as part of the habitual and total way in which we react to everything. This is generally developed before we are of an age to prevent it happening and, therefore, accidental. Sufferers are victims, not blameworthy. However, only you can direct yourself – nobody else can do it for you. You can learn to do so in a different way, learn how to respond to the stimuli of life in such a way that you don't hurt yourself. If a symptom of your pulling down is headache, then, when you learn to stop pulling down, headache will be a thing of the past. Certainly, my colleagues in the Professional Association of Alexander Teachers will be delighted to help you say goodbye to headaches.

\*

This article is based on the more detailed 'Headaches and the Alexander Technique' by Ian Whaley, published by the Professional Association of Alexander Teachers. Details can be obtained from: The Secretary, PAAT, c/o Ian Whaley, 14 Kingsland, Newcastle-upon-Tyne, NE2 3AL; tel. 0191 2818032.

## REFERENCES

1.  D. J. Dalessio, 'A clinical classification of headache', in Harold G. Wolff, *Wolff's Headache and Other Head Pain*, 6th edn, OUP (NY), 1993
2.  Basmajian and De Luca, *Muscles Alive*, 5th edn
3.  Moore, Keith L., *Clinically Oriented Anatomy*, 2nd edn, pp. 879 and 1006; Green, J. H., and Silver, P. H. S., *An Introduction to Human Anatomy*, OUP, 1981, pp. 261 and 316
4.  L. Kudrow, 'Cluster headaches', in Wolff, ibid., chapter 7
5.  Empson, Jacob, *Sleep and Dreaming*, 2nd edn, Pentland Press, 1995

Abbey Brook Cactus Nursery
Dept CP
Bakewell Road
Matlock
Derbyshire DE4 2QJ

Sells the cactus *Cereus peruvianus*, which has been shown to absorb electromagnetic radiation from VDUs and televisions.

Action Against Allergy
Amelia Hill
43 The Downs
London SW20

AAA (Action Against Allergy) provides an information service on all aspects of allergy and allergy-related illness, free to everyone. Supporting members get a newsletter three times a year and a postal lending-library service. AAA can supply GPs with the names and addresses of specialist allergy doctors. It also has a talk-line network which puts sufferers in telephone touch with others through the NHS and itself initiates and supports research. Please enclose s.a.e. (9 × 6 in) for further information.

BioCare Ltd
54 Northfield Road
Norton
Birmingham B30 1JH
Tel. 0121 433 3727

Wide range of nutritional supplements for candida control and allergies including: Mycropryl (slow-release caprylic acid), Cystoplex (cranberry juice capsules), butyric acid complex (food allergies). Biocare is the only UK company in the practitioner market that manufactures its own range of Probiotics – live bacterial supplements to kill off harmful organisms in the gut – in its own facilities. BioCare's Bio-Acidophilus is the only Probiotic on the UK market derived from a research grant from the British Department of Trade and Industry.

British Holistic Medical Association
179 Gloucester Place,
London NW1 6DX

British Migraine Association
178a High Road
Byfleet
Weybridge
Surrey KT14 7ED

Cirrus Associates
Food and Environmental Consultancy
Little Hintock
Kington Magna
Gillingham
Dorset SP8 5EW;
Tel. 01747–838165.

A wide range of products including VDU screen protectors, allergy-safe kettles and cooking appliances. Advice on allergies and special diets.

Colonic International Association
14 Englands Lane
London NW3
Tel: 0171 483 1595

Family Health & Nutrition
PO Box 38
Crowborough
Sussex TN6 2YP

Federation of Aromatherapists
46 Dalkeith Road
London SE21

Health Plus Ltd
PO 86
Seaford
E. Sussex
BN25 4ZW
Tel. 01323 492096

Suppliers of convenient candida control pack and other products.

Herbs of Grace
Peter Enkel
5 Turnpike Road
Red Lodge
Bury St Edmunds
Suffolk LP28 8JZ
Tel. 01638 750140

Counselling on and supply of herbal remedies for migraine and
other health problems.

Institute of Allergy Therapists
Short courses in the diagnosis and treatment of allergic con-
ditions. The institute maintains a register of practitioners and pro-
vides a referral service for the general public. Write to: Donald
M. Harrison, BA (Hons), BSc, MR Pharm S, Institute of
Allergy Therapists, Ffynnonwen, Llangwyryfon, Aberystwyth,
Dyfed SY23 4EY.

Life Tools
Department SC 1
Sunrise House
Hulley Road
Macclesfield
Cheshire SK10 2LP

Suppliers of compact machine (Mind Lab) which works with
light and sound frequencies (light frames and earphones) to alter
brain wave patterns to promote relaxation and sleep, or raise
energy and concentration levels. Can be extremely effective for
tension headaches. Some migraine sufferers have found it beneficial after continued use. Initially there may be an increase in
symptoms. Contraindicated with epilepsy.

Available for fifteen–day trial (UK), longer overseas. (Comes with plug adaptor for country of use.)

Lifeline Natural Foods
Mail Order Service
42 Princes Street
Yeovil
Somerset BA20 1EQ

Migraine Trust
45 Great Ormond Street
London WC1N 3HD
Tel: 0171–278 2676

National Institute of Medical Herbalists
41 Hatherley Road
Winchester
Hants SO22 6RR

National Society for Research into Allergy
PO Box 45
Hinkley
Leicestershire LE10 1JY

New Nutrition
Penny Davenport
Woodlands
London Road
Battle
E. Sussex TN33 0LP
Tel: 01424 774103

Nutritional advice for all health problems; Health Letter service; telephone and personal consultations; send s.a.e. for details.

Nutrition Associates
Galtres House
Lysander Close
Clifton Moorgate
York YO3 OXB
Tel: 01904 691591

Medical practice: candida/allergy testing, nutritional profiles, full-spectrum lighting.

Nutrition Line, see New Nutrition

The Patients' Association
Room 33
18 Charing Cross Road
London WC2 OHR
Tel: 0171–240 0671

Pre-Menstrual Tension Advisory Service
PO Box 268
Hove
Sussex BN3 1RW

Counselling for candida and cystitis; also books and videos: phone Angela Kilmartin 0171–249 8664

Sanford Clinic
15 Lake Road North
Roath Park
Cardiff CF2 5QA
Tel: 01222 747507

Society for Environmental Therapy
3 Atherton Street
Ipswich
Suffolk IP4 2LD

Wholefood, organically grown produce
24 Paddington Street
London WIM 4DR

# INDEX

References to figures are in *italic*

acupuncture meridians, *195*

adrenalin, 27–8

  adrenal gland reflex, 227

alcohol

  and drugs, 106

  and hypoglycaemia

    behaviour, effect on, 144–5

    connection with, 141–2

    giving up, 142–4

    gradual withdrawal, 144

    nutritional supplements, 145–6

  migraine trigger, 70, 72

  muscle relaxant, 9

Alexander Technique

  benefits of, 234–6

  out of shape bodies, 232–3

  principle of, 231–2

  pulling down, 233–4

  relieving spine problems, 176

  resting, *178*

allergies

  allergic reactions, 99–100

  allergic rhinitis headaches

    case history, 108–9

    chemicals, 104–5

    drugs for, 105–8

    hay fever, 103–4

    inhaled substances, 104

  allergic sinus headaches, *see* sinus

  allergy headaches, 101–2

  antibodies, 100

  food and chemical intolerance, 100–101, 112–14

  immune system, role of, 100

  second exposure, 100–101

  testing, 86, 109–10

# READ MORE IN PENGUIN

In every corner of the world, on every subject under the sun, Penguin represents quality and variety – the very best in publishing today.

For complete information about books available from Penguin – including Puffins, Penguin Classics and Arkana – and how to order them, write to us at the appropriate address below. Please note that for copyright reasons the selection of books varies from country to country.

**In the United Kingdom**: Please write to *Dept. EP, Penguin Books Ltd, Bath Road, Harmondsworth, West Drayton, Middlesex UB7 ODA*

**In the United States**: Please write to *Consumer Sales, Penguin USA, P.O. Box 999, Dept. 17109, Bergenfield, New Jersey 07621-0120.* VISA and MasterCard holders call 1-800-253-6476 to order Penguin titles

**In Canada**: Please write to *Penguin Books Canada Ltd, 10 Alcorn Avenue, Suite 300, Toronto, Ontario M4V 3B2*

**In Australia**: Please write to *Penguin Books Australia Ltd, P.O. Box 257, Ringwood, Victoria 3134*

**In New Zealand**: Please write to *Penguin Books (NZ) Ltd, Private Bag 102902, North Shore Mail Centre, Auckland 10*

**In India**: Please write to *Penguin Books India Pvt Ltd, 706 Eros Apartments, 56 Nehru Place, New Delhi 110 019*

**In the Netherlands**: Please write to *Penguin Books Netherlands bv, Postbus 3507, NL-1001 AH Amsterdam*

**In Germany**: Please write to *Penguin Books Deutschland GmbH, Metzlerstrasse 26, 60594 Frankfurt am Main*

**In Spain**: Please write to *Penguin Books S. A., Bravo Murillo 19, 1° B, 28015 Madrid*

**In Italy**: Please write to *Penguin Italia s.r.l., Via Felice Casati 20, I–20124 Milano*

**In France**: Please write to *Penguin France S. A., 17 rue Lejeune, F–31000 Toulouse*

**In Japan**: Please write to *Penguin Books Japan, Ishikiribashi Building, 2–5–4, Suido, Bunkyo-ku, Tokyo 112*

**In South Africa**: Please write to *Longman Penguin Southern Africa (Pty) Ltd, Private Bag X08, Bertsham 2013*

# READ MORE IN PENGUIN

## A SELECTION OF HEALTH BOOKS

### Food for Thought  David Benton

There has been an explosion of interest in the possibility that what we eat affects our behaviour. *Food for Thought* steers a path through the sensational claims to a series of well-researched and sensible conclusions.

### Children First  Penelope Leach

Penelope Leach argues that society today leaves little time or space for children and no easy way for adults – especially women – to be both solvent, self-respecting citizens and caring parents. *Children First* is her call to action.

### Woman's Experience of Sex  Sheila Kitzinger

Fully illustrated with photographs and line drawings, this book explores the riches of women's sexuality at every stage of life. 'A book which any mother could confidently pass on to her daughter – and her partner too' – *Sunday Times*

### The Effective Way to Stop Drinking  Beauchamp Colclough

Beauchamp Colclough is an international authority on drink dependency, a reformed alcoholic, and living proof that today's decision is tomorrow's freedom. Follow the expert advice contained here, and it will help you give up drinking – for good.

### Living with Alzheimer's Disease and Similar Conditions
Dr Gordon Wilcock

This complete and compassionate self-help guide is designed for families and carers (professional or otherwise) faced with the 'living bereavement' of dementia.

### Living with Stress
Cary L. Cooper, Rachel D. Cooper and Lynn H. Eaker

Stress leads to more stress, and the authors of this helpful book show why low levels of stress are desirable and how best we can achieve them in today's world. Looking at those most vulnerable, they demonstrate ways of breaking the vicious circle that can ruin lives.

# READ MORE IN PENGUIN

## A SELECTION OF HEALTH BOOKS

**Infertility**  Elizabeth Bryan and Ronald Higgins

Positive and sympathetic, this book will guide infertile couples, questioning health workers and the concerned general reader alike through a maze of fascinating new issues involving medicine, technology, counselling, ethics, law and health economics. It frankly confronts all the painful medical and moral choices while celebrating dramatic new hopes for the childless.

**Mixed Messages**  Brigid McConville

Images of breasts – young and naked, sexual and chic – are everywhere. Yet for many women, the form, functions and health of our own breasts remain shrouded in mystery, ignorance – even fear. The consequences of our culture's breast taboos are tragic: Britain's breast-cancer death rate is the highest in the world. Every woman should read *Mixed Messages* – the first book to consider the well-being of our breasts in the wider contexts of our lives.

**Defeating Depression**  Tony Lake

Counselling, medication and the support of friends can all provide invaluable help in relieving depression. But if we are to combat it once and for all, we must face up to perhaps painful truths about our past and take the first steps forward that can eventually transform our lives. This lucid and sensitive book shows us how.

**Freedom and Choice in Childbirth**  Sheila Kitzinger

Undogmatic, honest and compassionate, Sheila Kitzinger's book raises searching questions about the kind of care offered to the pregnant woman – and will help her make decisions and communicate effectively about the kind of birth experience she desires.

**The Complete New Herbal**  Richard Mabey

The new bible for herb users. It is authoritative, up-to-date, absorbing to read and hugely informative, with practical, clear sections on cultivation and the uses of herbs in daily life, nutrition and healing.

# READ MORE IN PENGUIN

## A SELECTION OF HEALTH BOOKS

### Allen Carr's Easy Way to Stop Smoking

Allen Carr's unique method can help *you* to stop smoking. He uses no scare tactics, removing the psychological need to smoke while you smoke, and illustrates how stopping doesn't mean weight gain or psychological dependence: it feels great to be a non-smoker.

### Helping Your Handicapped Child   Janet Carr

Now fully revised and updated, this book explains how to follow step-by-step behavioural methods in all aspects of your child's development, from everyday activities like dressing and eating to resolving problems with bed-wetting. It also includes useful suggestions on achievements, rewards, setbacks and when and where to seek further advice.

### Endometriosis   Suzie Hayman

Endometriosis is currently surrounded by many damaging myths. Suzie Hayman's pioneering book will set the record straight and provide both sufferers and their doctors with the information necessary for an improved understanding of this frequently puzzling condition.

### The New Our Bodies, Ourselves
The Boston Women's Health Book Collective

To be used by all generations, *The New Our Bodies, Ourselves* courageously discusses many difficult issues, and is tailored to the needs of women in the 1990s. It provides the most complete advice and information available on women's health care. This British edition is by Angela Phillips and Jill Rakusen.

### Your Child's Emotional and Behavioural Development
Dr T. Berry Brazelton

From conception onwards children are constantly changing, growing and developing. This comprehensive book takes parents through each of the major milestones in their child's development and offers sensible, practical advice on how to manage difficulties.